HOW THE BRAIN
EVOLVED

ALAIN

PROCHIANTZ
HOW THE BRAIN
EVOLVED

McGraw-Hill, Inc.

New York St. Louis San Francisco Auckland Bogotá
Caracas Hamburg Lisbon London Madrid
Mexico Milan Montreal New Delhi Paris
San Juan São Paulo Singapore
Sydney Tokyo Toronto

English Language Edition

Translated by W.J. Gladstone
in collaboration with
The Language Service, Inc.
Poughkeepsie, New York

Typography by AB Typesetting
Poughkeepsie, New York

Library of Congress Cataloging-in-Publication Data

Prochiantz, Alain, 1948 –
  [*Construction du cerveau*. English]
  How the brain evolved. Alain Prochiantz
      p. cm. — (The McGraw-Hill *HORIZONS OF SCIENCE* series)
  Translation of: *La Construction du cerveau.*
  Includes bibliographical references.
  ISBN 0-07-050929-8
  1. Brain—Evolution. 2. Neurogenetics. I. Developmental neuro-
physiology. II. Title. III. Series.
  QP376.P68313 1992
612.8'2—dc20   91-40362

The original French language edition of this book
was published as *La Construction du cerveau*, copyright © 1989,
Hachette, Paris, France.
Questions de science series
Series editor, Dominique Lecourt

TABLE OF CONTENTS

INTRODUCTION

Among the latest, most active and most fruitful areas of research, of which there have been many in the biological sciences in the past 30 years, this is one of the most fascinating. We are on the eve of finding out how the brain "works." Of course, not until tomorrow will we be able to describe the eve fully.

Not only are we accumulating knowledge on the structure and workings of this organ which only yesterday was still considered as the body's "black box," not only are we making great strides in understanding the delicate chemistry through which it is able to control a good deal of our behavior; we are also sketching and delineating the process whereby the fertilized ovum eventually develops into a brain, that unusual organ whose extraordinary complexity—particularly in humans—seems until now to have defied our mental powers, those very powers of which it is considered to be the seat.

In concise and accessible language, this little book provides a progress report on what we now call developmental neurobiology, and lays out before us its exciting intellectual and social implications and prospects.

Developmental neurobiology is an integral part of the neurosciences whose rapid expansion Jean-Pierre Changeux recently described in a famous work as a true intellectual revolution: the neurological revolution. Is this revolution as significant as were the sweeping changes in physics early in this century, with the appearance of the theory of relativity and the launching of quantum mechanics? Perhaps it is too early to tell.

In any event, there is no doubt that—just as with the concepts of time and space, the structure of matter and the limits of our ability to know—some of the key notions of our understanding of the world have begun to waver, then to topple, with the onset and now with the blossoming of the neurosciences.

On the horizon, we can already discern in a new light serious and irreducible philosophical questions which, in this case, involve the nature of thought and language, the relation between nature and nurture (heredity and environment), the very notion of the individual, and the place of our species on the evolutionary scale. In both cases, it is obvious that basic research is bound to have applications which may transform not just our way of thinking but also our way of life, and which are arousing reactions that range from enthusiasm to anxiety.

As is often the case in modern science, the onset of this revolution was marked, elicited and promoted by the convergence of several avenues of research that had developed independently of each other: in chemistry, molecular biology, neurophysiology and embryology.

This theoretical cooperation, now well established, is giving rise to exchanges of questions, concepts, and methods. It produces material for congresses and publications that scan the life of the international scientific community. We should add that the rapid rate of these advances, on decisive questions, would be inconceivable without the emergence of new techniques of investigation and implementation: for example, we now have a whole series of reliable instruments and procedures for recording the electrical or biochemical activities of the brain during the performance of a rigorously monitored task; by means of positron-emission tomography, or PET scans, we can see the state of activity of a group of neurons within the skull; we know how to graft cells and how to transfer genetic material; new anatomical techniques have been created.

To assess the scope of the neurological revolution and to comprehend what is radically new about research on the developmental formation of the brain, it may be worth our while to turn our attention to the history of the research efforts that have preceded it. Despite what we still too often tend to believe when it comes to scientific advances, this history is not some sort of triumphal march in which the mind, through continuous fine tuning of its concepts and observations, manages to acquire a more complete and thorough view of its objective: in this case, the brain and the central and peripheral nervous systems.

This history, which is indeed one of progress, is actually a history of conflicts in which the mind is constantly at odds with itself in its ambition to apprehend the natural phenomena it seeks to master. To start with, the obvious fact we have just mentioned—namely that the brain and thought are intimately related—did not really become accepted until after a conflict that has lasted more than five centuries.

We should recall that Aristotle (in the 4th century B.C.), believed that the heart, source of all heat and all movement, center of the organism, was the seat of sensations, passions and intelligence. By virtue of the general axiom that "all things need a counterweight to reach a state of equilibrium and achieve the golden mean," he saw the brain as a cold organ whose principal function was to "temper the heat and turmoil that rule the heart." By virtue of the same axiom, he felt that there was a difference in the nature of the brain (cold) and the spinal marrow (warm). Finally, in accordance with his cosmogonic theses, he described the brain as being composed of water and earth.

This fantastic conception of Aristotle's not only had the backing of his reputation as a great philosopher but also that of his authoritativeness as an extraordinary observer of nature. In so doing, he deliberately took a view opposite to that of another conception advocated in its day by Hippocrates (end of the 5th century B.C.). The author of the treatise *On the Sacred Disease* (epilepsy) taught that the brain is the seat of sensation, the organ of movement and judgment. This conception was partly taken up again some decades later by Plato who, in *Timaeus*, also advocated the idea that the brain is a part of the marrow which, originally, "like a ploughed field, was to receive the divine seed."

It was not until Galen appeared (the physician and philosopher from Pergamum and friend of Marcus Aurelius) in the 2nd century A.D. that the Hippocratic thesis was confirmed. Through skillful experimentations on animals, Galen succeeded in demonstrating that the brain does, in fact, play the central role in controlling the body and mental activity. Galen did more: he made the first clear-cut distinctions, within the brain, between the cavities and ventricles, on the one hand, and the "substance" on the other, noting and emphasizing its resemblance to the nerves.

From then on, even though Aristotle's thesis continued to captivate many of the best minds until the 18th century, those who worked in this field directed their efforts to the description of the brain's structure. A second obvious fact began to gain acceptance, namely that this organ is not undifferentiated but organized.

Nevertheless, the result of these efforts was strikingly imprecise until almost the 19th century, despite the writings of Andreas Vesalius and Costanzo Varolius in the 16th century and those of the English anatomist Thomas Willis in the 17th century who gave full due to the role of the cortex in controlling behavior. This long period of darkness can certainly be attributed to the direct link, now well established, between this "dangerous organ" and the theological and philosophical question of the immateriality of the soul. Discussions of the brain smacked of heresy, as it were. People dared not get too close to the subject. And when Descartes referred to the *epiphysis cerebri* (better known as the pineal gland) as the link between body and soul, he was not speaking as a physiologist but as a metaphysician.

In addition to this "political" reason, there was another and more technical one. Niels Stensen, one of the clearest thinkers among the 17th century researchers, noted that this organ is quite refractory to morphological analysis. When the encephalon is extracted from the cranial cavity and laid on the dissecting table, it is soft and collapses. A medical historian neatly characterized it as "an indescribable viscus," and this appellation summed up the thinking of the anatomists of the period.

Therefore, long before scientists discovered the techniques necessary to harden and fix it without in any way damaging it, they preferred to turn their attention to the cranium, or skull, a much more solid structure; and the age-old tradition of "telling" the strengths and weaknesses of a person's character by examining the shape and arrangement of the cranial bones remained with us until the time of Johann Kaspar Lavater, who gave it the name "physiognomy."

In fact, it was not until 1810, when Franz Josef Gall published his *Anatomy and Physiology of the Nervous System in General and of the Brain in Particular*, that the science of the brain actually began. A new doctrine called phrenology was born: it attained a popularity so vast that it is difficult to imagine today. We now remember phrenology as being the first system to propose the theory of cerebral localizations. We should be clear about what is meant by localization: it involves identifying all the distinct parts in the brain as well as assigning a specialized function to each. With Gall, this assignment was very free as regards anatomical data, even though he was well versed in dissection. So far as he was concerned, the important point was the philosophical thesis that this doctrine made possible, namely, that human moral and intellectual qualities corresponded to the existence and exercise of distinct innate faculties found in the cerebrum.

Traditionally, the proponents of innatism (the predominance of inborn influences) were the spiritualists: they attributed this innateness to the substantiality of an immaterial soul. With Gall, innateness changed camps and, in the name of science, switched over to the side of materialism. It is understandable that it did not win the favor of the political and academic authorities at the time. Napoleon Bonaparte and Georges Cuvier were bitter opponents, and it fared no better under the Bourbons during the Restoration.

As naive as these convictions may appear today and as fanciful as Gall's list of the twenty-seven basic faculties which he localized in the brain may be, a line of research had been started. The localization he proposed for the function of language in the anterior lobes of the cortex would even be confirmed some years later by Paul Broca on the basis of psychopathological studies of aphasia. In the history of science, it is not so unusual for a wrong idea to engender a right one.

It has been said that the end of the 19th century, with the works of Gustav Theodor Fritsch, Eduard Hitzig, and Paul Flechsig, was the golden age of cerebral localizations. However questionable the applications that were immediately and hastily attempted may have been (lobotomy, as early as 1891!), these researches made it possible to map the brain scientifically.

Are the current studies in the functional anatomy of the brain and the nervous system an extension or even a confirmation of the phrenological tradition? The thesis of cerebral localizations certainly opened up the way for such investigations. Yet, we should point out that, going back to Gall's immediate successors, who were not his disciples, the meaning of the term localization had changed: they had given up the idea of ascribing all human behavior, from the simplest to the most elaborate, to particular regions of the cortex. For example, they no longer sought to circumscribe the area responsible for predation or the area controlling devotion! Today we are aware of the role of association areas that blur any rigid connection between region and function.

Let us not be too hasty in accepting the "myth of the precursor," all the more so since we further had to free ourselves of the notion of innateness that we had borrowed, or even snatched, from the spiritualist tradition. And this is a whole other story: that of the relations between embryology and genetics, with their repercussions on the theory of evolution. I will not labor the point: Alain Prochiantz, a neuroembryologist who heads an internationally renowned team at the Collège de France, has put into perfect perspective the recent and revolutionary discovery of the genes involved in the development of an organism (developmental genetics), which from this point on seals the alliance among these three branches of science. As we now know, this alliance, which scientists had been looking forward to since the beginning of this century, could not be forged concretely until the advent of molecular biology, which did not really begin to flourish until the early 1950s.

The admittedly tentative bottom line of this story is that although the development of the human brain indeed appears to be programmed genetically, more latitude, more play, has been introduced in the execution of this program than is the case in other species. This amount of play, which means that there is no strict genetic determinism, is an expression of epigenesis: through the stabilization of particular neuronal networks, every human individual has inscribed in the very structure of the brain his or her own singular history: affective, social, and cultural.

Other studies have confirmed this exceptional epigenetic component. The most spectacular involves the well-known case of the "Japanese brain." As we know, the Japanese use two systems of writing, *kana* and *kanji*, one virtually alphabetical and the other ideographic, like Chinese. It appears that each of these systems concerns a different cerebral hemisphere, the left for *kana* and the right for *kanji*. An individual who, as a result of a lesion of the left hemisphere, experiences difficulties in reading and writing *kana*, has no problems with *kanji*, and the opposite is true if the lesion occurs in the right hemisphere.

Beyond this particular illustration, the most telling lesson of developmental neurobiology is this: the trait that distinguishes the nature of humans from that of other animals is not strictly located in their innate part; rather, the fact is that in humans this trait is such that the innate leaves some measure of indeterminateness which opens the possibility for nurture (the environmental factors) to exercise a powerful influence on the performance of the program being transmitted. As a result, humans, more than any other animal species, can free themselves from the constraints of nature. In other words, people's nature consists in not having a nature in the same sense that other animals do.

This restores in proper perspective the speculations of sociobiologists who believed that observations by ethologists on the genetic bases of animal behavior could be transposed to human behavior. In so doing, they were blatantly disregarding the very character of human epigenesis in order to pass off a certain inegalitarian and competitive social order as natural.

This should make us cautious and even vigilant in regard to the analogies between brain and machine that have been given free rein in the recent past. Can the brain be assimilated to a supercomputer? Does a computer think like a brain, and will it be able to equal or even replace it because, some day soon, it may surpass it?

The developmental point of view, which is that of Alain Prochiantz, keeps him out of the way of the bitter debates that have started around these questions, at the crossroads of the neurosciences and artificial intelligence. But on occasion we detect that the researches he describes call for reflection along a very different line. We may well find that the cards have been reshuffled and that a brand new hand has been dealt.

If, in addition to demonstrating that there are permanent changes in the organization of the neuronal circuits, we consider that the brain is not separate and apart from the rest of the organism, if the blood-brain barrier we have all heard about is only a "porous" barrier, to use the author's words, and if the brain embodies cellular materials that have originated in other systems of the organism—then we must acknowledge that thought, whose seat is in the brain, affects the whole body; or, if we prefer, that thought is always already implicated in the entire organism. Therefore, we also think with our hands and even with our feet.

But under these conditions, we have to give up trying to reduce the brain to a machine and thought to a calculation, sophisticated as they may be: technological models of the brain, from the telegraph to the computer, have always been based on such reductions.

I find it interesting that it is a developmental biologist who has come to speak of Freud with some favor, and who proposes a nonaggression pact to the psychoanalysts, without any ulterior motive of annexation. No matter what the future may hold for the startling interpretation of analysis that he gives us (no doubt with a touch of humor), the important point is that an appropriate place is left in the thought process for the world of fantasy and for free individual expressions that involve the body and the emotions.

Alain Prochiantz challenges reductionism in biology, rejecting the contemporary equivalents of the well-known formula enunciated in 1801 by Georges Cabanis: "the brain secretes thought like the liver secretes bile." But his criticism is leveled implicitly against every other reductionism, and notably computer science.

The conception of the brain presented here opens up to the thought process a prospect in which risk is the only norm, the only "ethics" against any and all conformity. If philosophy may be defined as thoughts about thought, philosophers who pay any attention at all to the work of scientists and who, for all that, have retained some taste for risk, ought not to remain indifferent.

Dominique LECOURT

I

WHAT IS

A BRAIN?

THE STRUCTURE OF THE BRAIN

In the past few years, there have been spectacular developments in the study of the brain. This is related to advances in the neurosciences, that is to say, to all of the investigations into the central nervous system and the peripheral nervous system from the standpoint of their structure, genesis, and impact on behavior. The concepts and techniques of molecular biology, combined with those of the branches of anatomy and physiology, have played a decisive role in the rapid rise of the neurosciences since the early 1960s. None of the descriptions of the cerebral organ we are now able to give would have been possible with such precision without their help.

The brain is reputedly one of the most complicated organs. This reputation is no doubt deserved, even if the notion of complexity is not univocal. Whether or not this is so, the brain plays a decisive role in animal behavior, from the simplest to the most elaborate.

Let us take as an example the fairly common practice of writing a page on the typewriter. The eyes follow the text. The pictures of the letters are first recorded on the cells of the retina and then conveyed in the form of electrical and chemical signals to an initial cortical relay nucleus in the thalamus, and then to the visual areas situated behind the cortex. This first stage is, as we see, essentially sensory.

Through connections between these sensory areas and other areas localized more frontally in this same cortex, the reader makes sense of the words being read. Furthermore, orders are sent to the muscles, those of the eyes, allowing the reader to follow the text; other orders are sent to other muscles, in this case in the fingers, so that the reader can type. Therefore, the sensory and interpretative work is succeeded by motor work.

Let us now imagine that the reading of this text evokes a memory; the reader may, as the occasion arises, become lost in a daydream, to the point where he or she may even stop working. This memory and daydreaming episode involves the activation of other regions of the brain.

This extremely simplified example illustrates two notions that are now clearly established. The first is that there are specialized areas in the brain: the sensory cortex (visual, auditory, olfactory, etc.); the cortex associated with cognition or emotion; the motor cortex; the subcortical regions that may serve as relay stations between the sensory or afferent fibers and the motor or efferent fibers; finally, regions more closely associated with various forms of behavior (feeding, sexual behavior) through the release of hormones. The second notion is that such cerebral localization is doubly innervated by multiple systems connecting the different regions. Thus, on the one hand, we have neural pathways that transmit sensory impulses from the periphery to the center and motor responses from the center to the periphery; and, on the other hand, neural pathways that interconnect all the different regions in the brain, so to speak.

These pathways are made up of specialized cells called neurons. Neurons, like all other cells in the organism, have cell bodies. But in addition, they possess specialized projections called dendrites and axons that are in contact with the dendrites and axons of other neurons at points called synapses. Sometimes, these synapses connect a nerve fiber and a non-neural cell of some other system, such as a muscle cell. Also, these neuronal projections may be very long, such as the ones connecting the motor neurons of the spinal cord to a finger muscle (up to about 3 feet long in humans). Sometimes, they are very short, as in the case of the neurons involved in local networks so called, which in the cortex process information (for example, a sensory message) locally.

Those specialized points of interaction between nerve cells that we call synapses are very numerous:

each neuron may have thousands of them. Furthermore, not all synapses are of the same type. Their differences are due in part to the structure of the signal released in the synaptic cleft—that is to say, in the space separating the area from which the chemical signal is released (the presynaptic portion) from the receptor area where it binds (postsynaptic portion). This signal is transmitted through what is known as a neurotransmitter or chemical mediator, because it has a mediating function: it alters the activity of the postsynaptic cell and, for example, causes a contraction of the muscle fiber located at the "exit" of the synapse, according to the activity of the presynaptic fiber, that is, the conduction of the nerve impulse in the motor neuron.

However, the complexity of the brain is not simply a result of this functional anatomy that has just been briefly outlined. There is yet another complexity which is due to the different types of cells constituting the brain. In addition to the neurons and their extraordinary variety of chemical, morphological, and connective characteristics, the nervous system includes non-neuronal cells that play a very important part in the development and functioning of the brain. The extraordinary diversity of the types and forms of these cells was described at the beginning of this century by the Spanish histologist Santiago Ramón y Cajal, whose work is still a standard in present-day anatomy.

These supporting cells are called glial cells or
neuroglia. This name, given to them in the 19th century by Rudolf Virchow, means "which glues the
neurons together." They include macroglia and microglia. The microglia, discovered early in this century
by Pio del Rio Hortega, a student of Ramón y Cajal,
have not yet been studied extensively. Still, we do
know that they are a part of the immune defenses of
the brain and help to eliminate dead cells, particularly
dead neurons. The macroglia are better known. The
two principal types of macroglia in the brain have
been given names suggested by their particular
shapes: oligodendrocytes (branched) and astrocytes
(star-shaped).

The oligodendrocytes (oligodendroglia) wrap
around the axons of certain neurons and produce a
complex chemical structure, myelin, whose function
is to insulate electrically each fiber that is ensheathed
(myelinated). The result of this electrical insulation is
to increase considerably the velocity of nerve impulse
propagation along the axon.

Astrocytes have a very different function. During the process of development and perhaps also in
the adult, more particularly when an injury occurs,
they synthesize the molecules that promote the plastic
(or repair) processes: cell division, cell migration,
growth of axons and dendrites, formation of synapses,
etc. But in addition to promoting repair, the astrocytes
act as buffer cells that keep the chemical environment

of the neurons constant, particularly by reabsorbing the potassium released during electrical activity of nerve cells.

FROM THE EGG TO THE BRAIN

From this brief description of the brain, the first thing we note is the extremely great diversity of its molecular and cellular components. But we also realize how truly infinite are the possible combinations for the formation of the neuronal circuits that form the basis of animal behavior. Such is the complexity of the cerebral organ. This complexity not only opens up a vast avenue of research to determine its components and structures, but raises a powerful and fascinating question: how is this single structure, whose molecular, cellular, and connective diversity is practically limitless, produced from a few cells that emerge from the division of the fertilized egg to form the rudiments of the nervous system?

In short, how do you make a brain from an egg?

Let us now look at this process of development. First, we note that it has a temporal dimension, that it occurs in sequence, each stage prepared by the previous stage either according to strict determination or based on a range of possibilities among which a choice is made under the influence of the environment. This is why we cannot discuss the formation of the brain

26

without touching, if only very briefly, upon the stages that lead from the fertilized egg to the rudimentary nervous system.

The strategies of development at work in different species are not the same. Here, we will take as our model the egg of a vertebrate amphibian, the African toad called *Xenopus*. However, for those who are really only interested in the human species, we should point out that the lines along which these two vertebrates develop are not very different in their principles, at least in these early stages. The most notable difference is that mammals produce extraembryonic appendages that enable the embryo to attach itself to the maternal uterus and to derive its nourishment from the mother.

After it is fertilized by the sperm, the egg begins a period of cell divisions called the cleavage period. It leads to the formation of a ball of cells resembling a mulberry, hence its Latin name of *morula*.

The cells of the *morula* continue to divide but leave a cavity inside the ball. To mark this stage of development, it is given the new name of *blastula*, from the Greek word for germ or bud. The cavity produced inside the ball is known as the *blastocoele*.

Are all of the blastula's cells equivalent? Are some of them already differentiated or at least in the process of differentiation? This question has given rise to a great deal of controversy that still has not quieted down entirely. However, there are two points that can fairly safely be made. First, not all cells are the same, and hence they are differentiated; and this differentiation depends on the location of each of these cells in the blastula. Second, despite this initial differentiation, most of the differentiation pathways are still reversible at this stage.

As Lewis Wolpert, a great contemporary embryologist, cleverly put it, the next stage is considered the most important in the history of the individual: more important than birth, marriage, or death. This stage, called gastrulation, is given over to the formation of the three initial layers from which all tissues of the adult organism are derived, including those of the central nervous system: the brain and the spinal cord. Starting inward and proceeding outward, these three leaflets are the entoderm, the mesoderm, and the ectoderm. The nervous system develops from the ectoderm. Although we cannot go into detail on the subject of this very complex process of formation, one of its aspects should be discussed because it has a direct bearing on the makeup of the brain.

The cells that will give rise to the rudiment of the future brain are situated in the dorsal (back) part of the hollow ball known as the blastula. These cells belonging to the primitive ectoderm may already be undergoing partial neural differentiation; however, their definite differentiation will not take place until they come in contact with another region, one of mesodermal origin. This contact between the primitive dorsal ectoderm and this region of the mesoderm constitutes the inductive signal for the formation of the primordial nervous system. The primitive ectoderm of the ventral (front) part of the blastula, which normally does not produce a nervous system, may be induced to differentiate into a nervous system if we artificially place it in contact with the inductive mesodermal region. The larva will then have two nervous systems. One of the great discoveries in the embryology of the nervous system is the identification of this inductive property of the mesodermal region. For this discovery we are indebted to two German embryologists, Olivia Mangold and Hans Spemann (1930).

Laboratories of molecular embryology have been investigating the chemical nature of this inductor since the end of the 1930s. However, we should not conclude that discoveries can be so easily programmed, because we still have no complete explanation, on a molecular level, of the mechanism of neural induction.

The rudimentary nervous system definitely appears in the next embryonic stage which, for this very reason, is called neurulation. By now, the embryo is elongated, and we can distinguish the positions of the future head and tail. The dorsal ectodermal part forms a cavity over the entire length of the embryo: the neural groove; this groove closes and forms the neural tube. During the closure of the tube, cells escape on either side and form the neural crests. They eventually migrate in the organism and become the ganglia of the peripheral nervous system. As for the neural tube, it will form the central nervous system, with the brain vesicles (rudiments of the different brain segments) to the front (endbrain, between-brain, midbrain, hindbrain) and the spinal cord to the rear, extending along nearly the entire length of what we may now call a tadpole.

As we see, the central nervous system resembles a tube, a hollow organ containing a fluid called the cerebrospinal fluid that circulates from the front (first cerebral ventricle) to the rear (last segments of the spinal cord). Therefore, what we call the brain is the product of a differentiation of the walls of the forwardmost (rostral) region of this tube. This anterior region itself appears to be segmented into a number of vesicles.

The first vesicle (endbrain) will give rise to the cortex and its different regions (sensory areas, motor areas, association areas, cognitive areas) and also to the subcortical nuclei involved in motor control and certain memory processes. The next vesicles will produce other regions of the brain which will not be discussed in any detail here.

However, it is important to understand that the fate of groups of cells is dictated at this stage by their position along the axes of the brain, exactly as in the previous blastula stage, the fate of cells was dictated by their position along other axes. Thus, positional information plays a major part in the processes of differentiation and morphogenesis. A distinction must be made between morphogenesis, the development of the shape of organs, and cell differentiation, that is, the mechanisms whereby a cell becomes, for example, a neuron or a glia cell.

We have just discussed the general framework of the development and organization of the brain as seen by the current neurosciences. There is an infinite number of questions that we could explore in this area. We will discuss some of them, perhaps the most important, in relation to the embryogenesis of the brain.

SOME QUESTIONS

Before discussing the type of researches now being conducted in this connection, we will now indicate which particular questions, in our opinion, are the essential ones.

As mentioned earlier, the cells that will eventually become part of the nervous system are of ectodermal origin. After differentiation, they give rise to the neurons, astrocytes, and oligodendrocytes. Thus, the first questions have to do with the genealogy of the different cell types: what are the signals responsible for the commitment of the cells to these different avenues of differentiation, and what are the family relationships among the three categories of cells?

31

For example, to take the case of the astrocytes and oligodendrocytes, we can conceive that there is an undifferentiated cell (stem cell) that divides into two daughter cells, one becoming an oligodendrocyte and the other an astrocyte. The two cells would then be sisters. But we can also imagine that the astrocytes are formed first, and that some of them divide and become differentiated into oligodendrocytes. In this case, they would be mother and daughter rather than sisters.

These very important questions define the bounds of the ongoing researches into the family relationships among the different cell types, or, to use a more technical term, into cell lineage. They encompass not only genealogical but also mechanical aspects, namely, an understanding of the mechanisms whereby a cell becomes differentiated. The difference between two cells (an astrocyte and an oligodendrocyte, to return to the same example) depends on the expression of a different set of genes for each cell type. In order to understand why a certain gene is expressed in a certain cell at a particular time during differentiation, we must first elucidate the mechanisms regulating gene expressivity. Despite the many advances made along these lines, we are still far from having a fully detailed understanding of these mechanisms.

Another question: the division and death of neurons. One of the characteristics of neurons is that they lose their ability to divide very rapidly. Unlike other types of cells, once neurons have become differentiated, they are no longer able to divide, barring rare exceptions (such as certain neurons involved in the sexual behavior of birds). Therefore, the total number of neurons in adults will depend on two factors: the cell division of their precursors during embryogenesis, and the death of neurons, during the course of aging, to be sure, but especially during embryonic development. Neuronal death is one of the major occurrences in the formation of the nervous system: depending on the regions of the system, from 10 to 80% of the neurons die during embryogenesis of the brain. The mechanisms of and reasons for this neuronal death is another burning issue in embryological investigations of the nervous system.

This is one of the points we will examine: during development, the brain cells, like all cells in the organism, undergo intense migratory activity. The mechanisms of migration as well as the phenomena that determine the pathways of migration are currently being studied.

But the nerve cells, those still migrating or the ones that have just completed their migration, are already lengthening their axons, those cell processes through which they come into contact with each other to form neuronal networks. This growth of axons and formation of the first contacts with the target sites, namely, the structures they innervate and where they establish synaptic contacts, raise different questions. What are the factors that induce the formation of projections, axons and dendrites? How does the projection find its way through the three-dimensional space of the brain matter? How does it recognize the cell with which it has to establish contact? How does it regress and disappear if contact is not made? To what extent are these contacts strictly determined and to what extent does chance come into play? These questions are all at the heart of developmental neurobiology.

We now recall our earlier reference to the extreme diversity of neuronal types, in contrast to the apparently monophyletic cell types after the formation of the neural tube. The question is of course determined by the signals through which a given neuron will synthesize a particular neurotransmitter rather than another. We do not know the answer as regards the brain, but we do have parts of the answer with respect to the peripheral nervous system. There, a molecule has been discovered that changes the type of mediator synthesized by certain neurons. As a result, we have an idea of the mechanisms through which a given neuron synthesizes a particular neurotransmitter.

To pursue this diversity, let us also recall that we previously mentioned glial cells in this regard: the microglia and macroglia. What we need to understand is not only how a particular cell is produced but also the physiological reason behind it. What is the purpose of the astrocytes, oligodendrocytes, and microglia? What is the structure of their interactions with the neurons? How can this multicellular whole be integrated into functional units? As we see, there is no dearth of questions.

Out of this inexhaustible list, here is one last question which we now propose to consider in some detail because it opens up an entirely new field of research and involves extremely important theoretical and practical considerations. This question relates to the determination of the localization and *form of the cerebral organs*, the constitution of their different regions and their differentiations in various animal species. It appears that we are on the verge of understanding the genetic mechanism of this morphogenesis. In any case, it will require the joint efforts of embryology, the neurosciences, and molecular biology to formulate clearly the question that has been posed. By taking a detour which will momentarily lead us out of the realm of the neurosciences in the strict sense of the term, we will try to present it in the simplest possible way.

II

THE GENETICS OF

CEREBRAL DEVELOPMENT:

HOW CLOSE ARE WE?

GENESIS AND EPIGENESIS

We must bear in mind that there is a particular historical and theoretical link between embryology and the neurosciences: indeed, for a very long time, the make-up of the nervous system was one of the most important models in the very development of experimental embryology. Let us remember Spemann, to whom we have already referred, and the question of neural induction as it was analyzed in the early days of this branch of science. This was the question to end all questions, the one around which embryology itself is built: from a single cell, how do we get several different types of cells? Spemann pondered this question: how does a cell which at the outset is undifferentiated eventually become a cell of the nervous system? Through what chemical or cell interaction mechanism is it induced to become, for example, a neuron? In other words, how is it that a cell, while endowed initially with a number of possibilities for differentiation, is led in the direction of becoming a nerve cell rather than, let us say, a muscle cell?

Such are the links between embryology and the study of how the nervous system develops: the study of the development of this system has provided embryologists with an opportunity to formulate in clear terms the concept of induction, which plays a central role in experimental embryology. As noted earlier, the primitive dorsal ectoderm of the blastula does not really differentiate into nervous tissue until after it comes into contact with the mesodermal layer during gastrulation. The necessity of this contact gave rise to the idea that differentiation must be induced.

However, with the emergence and then the extraordinary achievements of molecular biology in the late 1950s, new and extremely promising developments became possible and reorganized the relationship between embryology and nervous system research.

Before we explore these developments, let us take a moment to consider the investigations and concepts of those embryologists who worked between 1890 and 1950, that is to say, before genetics as such found its molecular bases. These concepts arose from a debate that lasted all the way through the 18th and 19th centuries and which is described in the collective work edited by Georges Canguilhem, *Du développement à l'évolution au XIXe siècle* [From development to evolution in the 19th century]. The theory of preformation, that is, the involution or incasement of germ cells, had been proposed in the 18th century by Charles Bonnet. According to the preformationists, the new being existed in a fully preformed state in the ovum (according to the ovists) or in the sperm (according to the animalculists or spermists), and embryonal development was only an enlargement (in the photographic sense) of all the organs of the *homunculus*. In turn, this *homunculus* had germ cells containing other *homunculi*, and so forth. Hence, the term incasement of germ cells given to this theory.

This theory was opposed by the 19th century embryologist Kaspar Friedrich Wolff, who demonstrated scientifically that the development of the different parts of the organism takes place through successive additions and differentiations from the ovum and then from a small number of undifferentiated cells. Wolff's concept formed the basis for a certain radical form of epigenetics.

Edouard Balbiani (1823–1899) may have been the first to point out that although embryogenetic research is consistent with the epigenetic description given by Wolff, there is a material principle passed on from generation to generation that is responsible for the fact that a chicken egg will produce a chicken and a duck egg will produce a duck, regardless of the conditions in which incubation take place. Therefore, this inherited material principle is responsible for the general form of the organism, or for its plan.

Thus, through the 19th century, the idea that two nonexclusive parts were involved in the fashioning of the organ systems made headway, although not without a good deal of difficulty: the first part is governed by strict hereditary determinism, and the second by intervention of the environment in the fashioning process.

Nature has provided a classic illustration of the existence of these two parts. In a given organism, let us take the case of twins who are genetically absolutely identical: the structure of their nervous systems should also be absolutely identical if the process of their development were governed solely by strict genetic determinism. On the contrary, we find in fact that in most organisms, two individuals who are absolutely identical genetically will never have identical nervous systems: whether we look at the number of nerve cells or at the network of their connections, we will find appreciable differences.

Therefore, there is flexibility within genetic determinism, and these variations between identical individuals are due to everything that can be called epigenetic—that is to say, everything that is not strictly determined by genes, everything that introduces some latitude around genetic determinism; this is indicated by the Greek prefix epi, which signifies something that is added onto, comes after, or is attached to, as well as the curve of a trajectory.

Nowadays, we know more about how the genetic and the epigenetic components share in development of an organism. In particular, by analyzing the different species, we have come to understand that the potential for plasticity, that is, for the capacity of an organism to vary in developmental pattern according to the history of the individuals, is greater as we "ascend" the scale from lower to higher animals: for example, epigenesis is a greater factor in vertebrates than in invertebrates.

The more evolved the species we are working with (say, mammals among the vertebrates), the greater the role of epigenetic mechanisms in the structure of the nervous system. In short, the higher we ascend, the less mechanical we become. I am using the word "ascend" because we know that the branch of vertebrates appeared historically after the invertebrate branch. I also use it for other reasons I shall mention in presenting the concept of evolutionary scale. For the time being, let me just point out that with the distinction between the genetic and the epigenetic, we have a basic distinction enabling us to shed light on the process of how the brain evolved.

Of course, this distinction applies to the whole organism; therefore, before we come to the brain itself, we should recall how today's research can help us look at the old question of embryology. From a single cell, the egg, how do we eventually reach organisms or individuals composed of a very large number of cell types (about two hundred) endowed with different properties? For example, a cell that proceeds to "fashion" a muscle, a nerve cell, a skin cell?

CELL DIFFERENTIATION AND TISSUE MORPHOGENESIS

The first process to consider in order to explain this prodigious mechanism is the process of cell differentiation that we mentioned in our description of the brain. From a cell, the egg, different divisions are formed. At a given time, the dividing cells will become nerve cells, muscle cells, etc. In other words, successive "decisions" are made during cell division, as a result of which a cell will acquire properties that will turn it into a neuron, for instance. These decisions can generally be pinpointed in time; they correspond to very specific moments. However, we should point out that a cell that is induced to make such a decision can turn back away from it for some time: there is a "window" during which the induction events remain reversible; after that time, in most cases, they become irreversible.

In these decisions, we are dealing with events resulting from interaction between the cell and its environment that are the stable expression of a given genetic repertory. Therefore, they are sequences of events that decide the fate of a cell, though the choice it is given is always a function of its previous history, starting with the egg.

We see that through a cascade series of steps the different possibilities available to the cell are gradually restricted until such time as it is assigned to the manu-

having a general application: involved here are the size and shape of organs. Let us suppose that overnight we have, for example, two additional divisions in a particular region of the brain during the development of an animal; this region will, of course, be larger in the mutant than in the normal animal. We can therefore say that developmental genes determine all at once the number, shape and, above all, arrangement of the cells that leads to the formation of a design for the organism.

Let us return to our *Drosophila* example to clarify what we mean today by a developmental gene. In the fly and especially in the maggot, segments immediately appear (like the segments in an earthworm) that follow each other in a sequence from the mouth to the anus. We should point out right away that while such segmentation is not quite a general occurrence (there is no segmentation in one-celled organisms or in organisms with radial symmetry such as sea urchins), it is at least very widespread. In vertebrates, the stacked-up arrangement of the vertebrae shows traces of such segmental origin.

We need not go into great detail discussing every step of the development of *Drosophila*. We need only point out that the position of the front and the rear, the dorsal region or the ventral region, the number of segments, the polarity of the segments (where is the front and where is the rear of each segment?), and the nature of the segments (does it carry a foot or an antenna?) are under genetic control, which means that there will be mutants whose front will be transformed to become the rear, producing a being with two caudal parts (bicaudal mutant) or mutants with two dorsal parts and no ventral part, or shortened mutants lacking a number of segments, or else mutants with a normal number of segments but having a segment that develops as if it were a different segment; for example, the head segment will develop as if it were partly thoracic, with the antenna transformed into a foot.

We can see immediately that so far as the morphogenesis of organs is concerned, the class of mutations we have just described answers the question we have raised. The same cells that should have produced one organ produced another one instead. It is not the nature of the cells that changed, they are still fibroblasts, nerve cells, muscle cells, etc.; what did change as a result of the mutation is the plan of organization, the construction pattern. Therefore, there are genes involved in controlling the form as derived from all of the cell interactions. These genes have been called homeotic genes because they transform an organ that is specific to a segment (the antenna for the head) into the homologous organ of another segment (the foot for the thoracic segment).

But can what we find in *Drosophila* also apply to other organisms such as vertebrates and humans? Let us begin by saying that homeotic mutation—that is, the transformation of one organ into another, homologous organ—was observed as far back as 1913 by Edwin Goodrich in sharks. Moreover, it has also been observed in humans. Without going into all the details, we can point out that the existence of families in which individuals have six fingers or more than one set of nipples, a not uncommon occurrence, is an instance of homeosis.

But let us return to the brain. How is it affected by homeosis? Formed during the neurulation stage, as we recall, is the neural tube, which runs through the dorsal region of the future tadpole from front to rear. The brain will be situated in the front with its different vesicles, the telencephalon, diencephalon, mesencephalon, rhombencephalon. The fate of the cells constituting the wall of the tube that will form the brain is partly dependent on their position. This suggests the following question: in the shaping of the different regions of the brain, can we conceive of a role for genes similar to the developmental genes and more precisely to the homeotic genes? Since the organ appears segmented and since the segments appear different, we are tempted to attribute such segmentation and such morphogenesis to the activity of these genes.

We must admit that even now there is still no proof that homeotic genes play a major role in this segmentation. In fact, there is not even proof that the brain is a segmented organ. It is not inconceivable, for example, that the apparent segmentation and the differences among segments are a consequence of the segmentation and differentiation of other tissues under homeotic regulation. For instance, we can imagine that segmentation affects the mesoderm surrounding the brain and that, by some indirect effect, the organ appears segmented. This would mean that the segmentation of the central nervous system is not the result of developmental gene expression in the brain cells themselves.

Nevertheless, as we must acknowledge, certain data suggest that homeotic genes play a role still poorly understood in the development of the brain. The best indication that this may be the case comes from molecular biology. It has been found that a nucleotide sequence (DNA is made up of nucleotides) was very often present in the homeotic genes of *Drosophila*, so much so that it was believed that this sequence called homeobox identifies a gene as being homeotic. Using molecular biology techniques, a search was made for this and for related sequences in vertebrates, in mammals, in humans—and they were found.

Even better, as regards the subject of immediate concern to us here, they were found in the nervous system, and even in the brain, in precise regions of the brain that may not correspond to segments but are clearly defined and therefore constitute distinct areas. There is much to be accomplished between the time that such genes are discovered in the brain and the moment when a specific function can be assigned to them with certainty. But this whole hypothesis has been postulated and the scientific literature is there to prove it. And if it should prove to be true, and if as a result we were able to understand how the different regions of the nervous system are organized, we would then have the key, the pattern for the structure: we would know why and how such and such a region is responsible for a given function: the cerebellum here, the cortex there, the mesencephalon over there. Yes, we would hold the major genetic key to the structuring of the brain.

This knowledge would be of many-faceted interest, but one of the main advantages would be to gain a new understanding of the phenomena of evolution: why it is that in some species, certain well-demarcated regions of the nervous system and the brain are more important than others. For example, the area related to the sense of smell is much more important in dogs than in humans; why, by contrast, are the structures related to cognitive functions more important in the human than in the chimpanzee? Even though the general pattern is the same in all vertebrates, not only are there modifications in the size of the cerebral organ, but also, within that organ, there are obvious differences between the regions that are more or less specifically involved in the exercise of a given function.

From the standpoint of species evolution, this would open the way to interesting animal experimentation. The creation of new species would be not just conceivable but achievable. We will now explore one of the prospects for such research by returning first to the questions of cell lineage, neuronal death, and the synthesis of neurotransmitters, which we put aside after describing the conditions in which they arose.

III

FROM CELL LINEAGE

TO THE CREATION

OF NEW SPECIES

A FEW OF THE MAIN AVENUES OF BASIC RESEARCH

Let us, therefore, begin with one of the initial questions we touched upon in the first chapter, the question dealing with cell genealogy. The term genealogy clearly illustrates the problem at hand. All cells are derived from one and the same cell: the egg. Hence, despite their differences, they are related. To keep to our subject of the brain, we can ask the following questions: at what point and by way of what mechanisms is a cell assigned to the construction of the brain? For a cerebral cell, how will the cell type—neuron, astrocyte, oligodendrocyte—be decided? More specifically, in the case of a neuron for example, how will it be decided that a given neuron is to belong to a particular region of the brain or to synthesize a particular mediator?

The approach is to identify a cell or a small population of cells by means of a label, a sort of tag, that will be retained as long as possible, that is, be transmitted through successive divisions and differentiations. Thus, after marking, by means of the label we can follow the fate of the daughter cells, granddaughter cells, etc. This means that lineage studies are very much dependent on the development of marking techniques. The first markings were performed in 1929 by the German neuropathologist Oskar Vogt in particular, with the use of stains. In this way, regions of the blastula (therefore, at the pregastrulation stage) were marked, and "fate maps" were drawn up. These fate maps, as their splendid name tells us, made it possible to determine—on the basis of where these regions were located on the surface of the blastula—to which tissue the descendants of the stained cells would be assigned as a matter of priority.

But these staining techniques had two limitations: the labeling was of short duration and there was no proof that the label, by its very presence, did not alter the fate of the cells. Since then, other labeling techniques have been developed, such as the injection with a microsyringe of a stain or protein that can produce color reactions. These have led to remarkable results, particularly in the United States in the hands of Marcus Jacobson and his group who were able in this way to study the lineage of most of the cells of the *Xenopus* blastula. But here too, the limitations of the technique were obvious, the main one being that the label is diluted with successive cell divisions until it becomes undetectable after a finite number of divisions. Furthermore, the injection requires large cells, which immediately rules out experiments in birds or mammals.

The first truly reliable label for birds was introduced and used by Nicole Le Douarin in the 1960s and 1970s. This label was, so to speak, a gift of nature. Quail cells differ from chicken cells by the fact that the nucleolus, a structure of the cell nucleus, has some distinctive and unvarying characteristics. A quail cell can always be distinguished from a chicken cell. Therefore, if at a given time, some quail cells are transplanted to the nervous system of a chick embryo, the quail cells can always be found and identified at any subsequent stage in the development of the chick, so that we can tell what they have become: for example, a neuron or a glial cell. Using this technique, Nicole Le Douarin and her coworkers were able to establish the genealogy of the peripheral nervous system cells (and more broadly the genealogy of cells of the neural crest alluded to previously) as well as those of the immune system in the chick. The same type of studies are now under way in the brain.

Unfortunately, such natural markers do not exist for all species, and furthermore, as we explained earlier, cell transplantation in the embryo is not easy when we deal with mammals rather than birds. Therefore, some other means of introducing stable markers had to be found. These lineage studies are now possible thanks to molecular genetics. Through molecular biology techniques (which we will not discuss in detail), it is now possible to introduce into the genome of a cell or of a limited number of cells a gene readily identifiable through its product. Provided that the gene is introduced into the genome of the cell in a stable manner, it divides at the same time as the genome itself and can no longer be diluted by cell division, since each daughter cell carries one or more copies of the genetic marker.

We can therefore expect to have in the not too distant future a genealogical tree of the principal types of cells in the brain. It will be able to answer the following question, for example: are two neurons belonging to two different regions of the brain closer cousins than two cells of different types (neurons and astrocytes) located in the same region? This is equivalent to asking: does a precursor cell know to what region it belongs before knowing whether it will be a neuron or an astrocyte? Or else: in the cell migration processes, what is assigned first, the "zip code" or the cell type?

The ability of the brain, not only as a whole, but also in its specialized regions, to process information, to solve problems, to participate in mental and behavioral functions, is dependent of course on the number of neurons and synapses that these regions contain. It is easy to understand that when we have a neuronal precursor in a given region, the final number of neurons will depend on the number of divisions of the precursor as well as on the death rate of the neurons; as mentioned earlier, this neuronal death is a major phenomenon in the embryogenesis of the brain (and of the nervous system in general).

Insofar as cell divisions are concerned, the problem is not necessarily different from the problem facing any cell. Therefore, we will focus our attention on the study of the mechanisms that regulate cell division. In particular, we will look at certain genes, specifically cell oncogenes, those "normal" analogues of the genes carried by certain viruses that cause an uncontrolled proliferation of the infected cells and result in the development of tumors. Actually, the study of the role of oncogenes and the regulation of their expression in the nervous system is a very active branch of developmental neurobiology. In addition, numerous studies, related of course to the ones we have just mentioned, are devoted to the search for molecules (or factors) which, once they come in contact with the cell precursors and bind to them through specific receptors, stimulate cell proliferation.

As regards neuronal death, we must admit that we still know practically nothing about the mechanisms involved. There are a number of models of cell death, particularly in the immune system, because there we find a specialized type of cell (killer cells) that kills foreign or infected cells, for example. According to one model, killer cells recognize the cells to be killed. Having recognized them, they make them porous by creating holes on their surface and causing them to burst; according to another model, they trigger a suicidal process in the recognized cell. It will certainly be one of the goals of this new discipline called neuroimmunology to understand the mechanisms of neuronal death.

Lastly, we must not forget that aside from determining the size of the brain or the size of its different compartments, neuronal death is one of the means whereby the neuronal networks are selected epigenetically among a practically infinite repertory of possible networks. Without any doubt, learning ability is based partly on this property of neurons to die and not be replaced, as paradoxical as this may seem to anyone who necessarily associates learning with acquisition or growth.

During the formation of the brain, numerous events of a migratory nature occur. They include the travel of the neuroblasts from their germinal zone to their final location, and extension of the axons. The growth of the neuronal projections is due to the migration of a structure situated at their tip, called the growth cone. The cone advances and pulls behind it the neuronal fiber whose material is synthesized in the cell body. We can possibly liken this process to the way a spider or a silk worm pulls on its thread.

We can immediately think of a series of questions that arise in this connection.

What is the motor of this mechanism? How is the motion triggered (problem of the start) and what causes it to stop (stop signal)? Finally, there are the problems of guidance in the three-dimensional space of the brain. How is a cell or a growth cone guided toward its destination? This is, of course, a crucial question, because the first step in the formation of the neuronal circuits depends on such guidance. To take a very schematic example, sight would be impossible if, instead of moving in the direction of the cerebral areas whose function is to process visual information, the growth cones of the ganglionic neurons of the retina headed for other regions of brain.

So far as the mechanical phenomenon of migration is concerned, our understanding of it is still incomplete. Several factors are involved, such as adhesion to the support made up of the other cells, and the ability of a cell or a growth cone to activate mechanisms of extension and contraction of cell expansions, somewhat like an arm that reaches out for support (extension) and then pulls the whole weight of the body behind it (contraction). These forces, in fact, are created by cytoskeleton proteins very similar to the proteins found in muscle fibers. This migration is possible only if the cells or the growth cone are capable of attaching to the support made up of the other cells; otherwise, there would be no point of support. Several types of molecules are involved in this attachment mechanism: some are called adhesion molecules, and others are molecules of the extra-cellular matrix.

The adhesion molecules are anchored in the cell membrane they cross, while the molecules of the matrix found outside the cells become attached through receptor molecules. These receptor molecules that cross the membrane are in contact with the molecules of the cytoskeleton (the motor).

Again, many questions arise and the answers are inconclusive. We need an inventory of all adhesion and matrix molecules as well as of the protein matrix receptors; we must also gain an understanding of their respective roles and analyze how the interactions among these proteins can result in movement. Finally, it is important to analyze these molecules and to determine the times they appear or disappear during development in order to understand why a given cell begins to migrate or stops migrating. That also applies to the growth cones.

One question of great interest relates to the way in which the cells or the growth cones guide themselves in space. In some cases, the question of directional response is predetermined by the fact that the very structure of the tissue surrounding the cell or the cone leaves no other choice but to follow a certain path (provided of course that the support permits migration processes to take place). However, we know from experience a second way to guide a cell: establishing a gradient of a molecule in relation to which the cell (or the cone) exhibits a positive tropism (for example, the sunflower has a positive tropism for sunlight). A molecule is said to be in a gradient position when its concentration varies between two given points.

Let us assume that cell B synthesizes a factor that diffuses in the medium and forms a concentration gradient, and that the cells characterized by a positive tropism for this factor will move toward B; this is called a chemotactic process. However, a third means of directional response, similar to the one just mentioned, has been discovered: in this case, factors bound to the growth substrate are used, and chemotaxis is replaced by haptotaxis. The best known chemotactic phenomenon involves a factor discovered in the 1950s in the United States by an Italian researcher, Rita Levi-Montalcini. This is the nerve growth factor (NGF).

NGF is a factor of survival, maturation, and axonal extension for specific classes of neurons, essentially certain neurons of the peripheral nervous system. The growth cones of these neurons can direct themselves along an increasing NGF gradient. Again, if we think of the large number of neurons of different types that are found in the brain, it is clear that the search for factors of survival, maturation, axonal extension, and spatial signalling, as well as the study of the mechanisms whereby these factors exert their action, is one of the most active sectors of research relating to the development of the brain.

The phenomena we have briefly described above are involved in the formation of neuronal circuits. However, we could say that they constitute only the general "package" or encompassing structure. We would like to emphasize at this point that questions also arise about the much finer circuits resulting from the synapse formation activity (synaptogenesis).

Synapse formation is one of the most important points in that, ultimately, the structure of the networks is determined by the distribution of synapses. As stated earlier, the synapse consists of a presynaptic cell that releases a chemical mediator (neurotransmitter) and a postsynaptic cell to which this neurotransmitter binds via a specific receptor. In the nervous system, there are different neurotransmitters and therefore different receptors.

This binding produces changes in the activity of the postsynaptic cell, from transient, rapid changes all the way to long-lasting changes (such as changes in genetic expression). These changes indicate that a message has been transmitted. To illustrate this point, we can refer to the contraction of muscle fiber which is produced by the binding of acetylcholine (a neurotransmitter released by motor neurons) to muscle cells. In the brain, the postsynaptic neuron does not contract, but its activity is modulated according to various modalities that will not be described here.

Once more, let us make it clear that the formation of synapses is of fundamental importance because, together with the forms of the neurons, it determines the structure of the networks that constitute the cellular basis of behavior. Therefore, learning, which is by definition a change in behavior, comes about through a change in the cell form, in the synaptic structure, or in the transmission effectiveness of the signal.

Hence, during the developmental formation of the synaptic network, the stage of recognition between the presynaptic cell and the postsynaptic cell—a stage that precedes the formation of the synapse—is essential. In some cases, and with certain species, it was assumed that this recognition was based on a purely genetic code. It is clear that such a mechanism, with the constraint that it implies, leaves little room for epigenetic plasticity and hence for learning.

This is why it is important that, within the framework of some genetic constraint, the formation of neuronal circuits, as is also the case with neuronal death, should leave something to chance. In fact, we do know that, at the start, the number of synapses in the process of formation is greater than the ultimate number, and that the final number is established during a selection process which involves a functional component that we may call learning. Let us recall the pithy aphorism of Jean-Pierre Changeux: "To learn is to eliminate."

The precise mechanism of this selection of neuronal circuits underlying all animal behavior and major body functions is obviously of the greatest importance. We will return to this question later, but it is only by understanding these rules of selection that we shall be able to apprehend scientifically the processes of individuation and plasticity that characterize the subphylum of vertebrates and, more than any other, the human species.

But the fact that the precise formation of the circuits and networks is based on a stochastic (or random) process which accounts for the acquired influences that help to shape the fine structure of the brain (identical twins will never have the same synaptic connections) does not obviate the fact that the general structure of the cerebral organ is dependent on the genome. The genetic potential characteristic of the species lays open the possibility for normal cerebral development, and the realization of that possibility depends on the history of the individual and his or her environment. Nevertheless, no matter how rich this environment may be, the genetic contents characteristic of the species set a limit beyond which one cannot go. No matter how often monkeys are placed in a human environment, they will never turn into humans as a result.

Therefore, one of the great challenges of neurobiology will be to discover which are the genes that determine, for instance, the size of the brain and of its different regions. For the time being, we have no indication of the nature of these genes. It is conceivable that by analyzing the genetic differences between closely related species (the chimpanzee and human, for example) or by further investigations into developmental genes (such as oncogenes and homeotic genes, though not exclusively), advances can be made in this area.

THERAPEUTIC APPLICATIONS

The work, past and present, whose main lines we are attempting to present briefly, is an important part of basic research in developmental neurobiology. It satisfies that cognitive curiosity built into the human cerebral structure and so participates in a learning function as natural to us as the function of nutrition or respiration; it does not have to be justified by any application. Nevertheless, applications already exist or can be anticipated in the foreseeable future: they carry hope for appreciable improvements in the human condition and for expansion of our knowledge in scientific areas outside of neurobiology. It would be impossible to describe all these applications, and I shall therefore confine myself to two areas: that of neurodegenerative diseases and cerebral aging, and the theory of evolution.

For example, let us take the repair of genetic defects, for instance in a disease where a key gene that synthesizes an important molecule is defective or missing. As of now, it is not inconceivable that cells in which such a gene has been implanted and rendered functional could be introduced into the diseased body, thereby repairing a genetic defect locally. This method is being seriously considered to treat Parkinson's disease.

We know that some forms of this disease are due to the premature death of neurons that play an important role in the control of motor activity and synthesize a particular neurotransmitter, dopamine. One of the current treatments is to administer a dopamine precursor which is converted to dopamine in the striatum, a region of the brain normally innervated by dopaminergic nerve endings.

The metabolism and seminal influence of dopamine was made known by laboratory studies of Julius Axelrod in the United States in the 1950s and the work of many other research teams. In particular, the gene that codes for the enzyme involved in the synthesis of dopamine has been reproduced in the laboratory. Therefore, this opens up the possibility of inserting this gene into cells in such a way that the enzyme will become active and dopamine will be secreted, and then introducing these cells into the striatum so that the necessary quantity of dopamine to repair the motor deficit would be "pumped out" continuously. Such a project is conceivable; it would first have to be carried out and tested as extensively as possible in animals before being applied to humans. This is an ethical question to which I will come back after considering another aspect of transfer and transplantation technology.

The technology incorporating the principle we have just mentioned combines a genetic procedure (gene transfer) and a physiological procedure (cell transplantation in the striatum). It is possible to dispense with the genetic stage by transplanting embryonal dopaminergic cells. Many of these techniques were developed by Professor Anders Björklund and his group in Lund, Sweden, and embryonal cells can now be implanted in the rat, the mouse, and even the chimpanzee, although few studies have yet been undertaken in that animal. In certain cases, these embryonal cells are found to become functional. This is the case, in particular, with embryonal neurons. They are able to synthesize and to release into the environment substances important to the nervous system, especially dopamine. Animal models of Parkinson's disease have, therefore, been devised: in these animals, usually rats, a chemical or mechanical procedure was applied to destroy the neurons that die in Parkinson's disease and whose death is responsible for the ensuing motor symptoms. By transplanting dopaminergic cells taken from rat embryos into the striatum, it has been possible to replace some of the dead neurons and to suppress certain of the behavioral disturbances.

Finally, it became possible just recently to reconstitute neuronal circuits, particularly by researchers working in the laboratory directed by Professor Constantino Sotelo at the Salpêtrière Hospital in

Paris. This time, reconstitution is no longer achieved by injecting a mass of cells to synthesize molecules which, when released in the brain, restore the operation of the machine, as if the gears have been oiled again. The procedure now is to restore precise synaptic connections in mutants which lack these connections because they are missing a neuronal population, especially in mutant mice whose cerebellum is deficient. Since we believe that many degenerative phenomena in the central nervous system are attributable to the death of specific categories of neurons, it might eventually be possible to repair certain brain impairments due to aging, whether normal or pathological, as in the case of Alzheimer's disease.

But from this opening that could lead to concrete treatments, the road is long and full of pitfalls. In fact, the use of animal models just mentioned raises a number of questions that cannot be ignored. We have seen the value of these models for research: to repair a deficit whose cause is precisely known since it is embodied in the very operation to which the animal selected had been subjected previously. These are indeed true experimental models. The question that then arises concerns transposition to humans: can we dispense with such models, as simplified as they may be?

Once again, Parkinson's disease is a particularly appropriate example for considering this question and weighing the serious stakes involved. We must note that attempts at random transplantation have been undertaken in recent years on patients desperate enough to agree to submit to this type of surgery. But we must recognize that at the present time we know almost nothing about the etiology of this disease: there is no reason, therefore, to think that the implanted cells might not be destined to die in exactly the same manner as the ones they were supposed to replace. Unfortunately, woeful failures have confirmed the suspected excessive haste, leaving the patients even more helpless.

An absolute prerequisite is to go through all the intermediate steps, such as the use of experimental protocols in the chimpanzee, for example. To operate directly upon humans in such a case is to risk not only an ineffective result but even more destruction than the disease process itself. May I add at this point that the intermediate steps include not just experimentation in animals but the development of basic research as well. It is not enough to transplant neurons and to say "growth is occurring" or "repair is taking place"; we must transcend the empirical context and determine why "growth is occurring" or "repair is taking place." Of course, that is more difficult and certainly less spectacular.

Some researchers, impelled by an ideology and a mode of financing that would make therapeutic application the only goal of research, blinded by the prospect of easy glory in the media, have, I feel quite free to say, played sorcerer's apprentice and have behaved at best as reckless individuals and at worst as dangerous lunatics or even criminals. Can we hope that scientists will draw a lesson from this, as well as—who knows?—the media which carry their share of responsibility in these matters?

I hope, in particular, that this will be the case with Alzheimer's disease, an early cerebral aging that destroys gradually, and sometimes rapidly, the intellectual functions of the individual. We now know which type of neurons degenerate first in the brains of persons afflicted with this terrible disease: the cholinergic neurons. Therefore, we have a right to be apprehensive that attempts will be made to transplant such neurons in the patients with the same disastrous haste as in the case of Parkinson's disease.

These are questions of medical ethics, one might say, or at least of deontological ethics; the regrettable excesses that have occurred are, I repeat, ascribable in part to a desire for hasty media publicity which has seized scientific and especially medical circles for a number of years now; they can be explained by the atmosphere of heightened international competition that surrounds certain types of investigations; they are linked, of course, and very directly so, to the huge financial stakes involved in the development of certain treatments. As we see, therefore, this ultimately raises very serious problems with regard to the structure of research financing and the relationship of research with what we have come to call society's needs, which should be identified: Who creates these needs? Who determines them? Who manipulates them? We will return to this in a little while.

But we cannot evade another question, which could be described as symmetrical, in connection with animal experimentation: it concerns the animals themselves. This question is not as trivial as it might appear. Of late, it has even become particularly acute. We have to see exactly what it entails and avoid being irrational.

The evolutionary scale, as we are aware, shows that between humans and other animal species, there is at the same time a continuity and a *radical difference*. The radical difference is due precisely to a development of cognitive functions distinctive of our species. Later on, we shall have occasion to draw some philosophical conclusions from this situation. Right now, however, we should point out that this question does have practical repercussions on research. For the past few years, we have witnessed a resurgence in public opinion and even among some eminent researchers of a particular form of spiritual values in defense of animals, which we could call animal spirituality.

Claude Bernard, in his day (1813–1878), already faced such problems. We know that before entering the Collège de France, when he used to conduct experiments in makeshift laboratories, he was often forced to move because of complaints from his neighbors. Not only was he accused of making the animals suffer, there was even a rumor that he secretly brought young children into his laboratory during the night in order to use them for experiments! Skipping over the anecdote of the police official's dog, let us just say that it was only through the protection of a kindly disposed and intelligent police captain that he was able to continue his research for two years. We also know that his wife was a militant antivivisectionist in an organization whose chairman was none other than Victor Hugo, and that she succeeded in pitting her daughters against their father over this issue. Even though this conflict was not the only cause of the affective solitude in which the scientist lived out his final years, it was partly responsible for it.

In his famous *Introduction à la médicine expérimentale* [Introduction to experimental medicine], Claude Bernard was indignant about the fact that the only use of animals condemned by those kind souls was medical research, even though, as he reminded us, its purpose is to find treatments to help human beings, while they uncomplainingly accept the castration of animals later to be butchered, a practice more difficult to justify.

We have referred to animal spirituality. It is really tantamount to disregarding the radical difference that separates humans from animals. In bringing the former down to the same level as other animal species, and in attributing a form of soul to dogs, mice, and pigs; why not tomorrow to *Drosophila* and bacteria? Thus, particularly in the English-speaking countries, perhaps because there is no Cartesian tradition ("the animal as a machine"), powerful organizations have been established with the self-appointed mission to defend so-called animal rights.

Let us be clear about this: we are not saying that everything and anything may be done to animals. Unnecessary suffering cannot be justified. I am thinking in particular of the mass torture practiced by certain cosmetic manufacturers when they use rats or rabbits to test the dermatological toxicity of their products for purely commercial ends. However, there are many instances in which no progress could be achieved in research without killing animals; and even, at the risk of shocking some, without causing them to suffer. Let us take, for example, as an extreme but very significant case, research on pain; we should not forget that the purpose of such research is to develop new drugs that will enable human beings to suffer less. Anyone who has witnessed the horrible pain that accompanies, for example, cancer at the terminal stage of the disease will immediately understand what is at stake.

To move from the specific area of neurosciences without leaving this difficult question, how could we not be surprised at the indignant hostility that was aroused after the recent announcement in England that it would be possible to transplant organs taken from pigs, hearts in particular, to humans; these reactions were not expressed according to some narcissistic logic that might see in this an affront to human dignity, but as an attack on the dignity of pigs! Are we about to relive, in reverse as it were, the great 17th-century quarrel about the soul of animals? Would this be a quarrel in which instead of viewing humans as animals in order to better understand them, we would humanize animals in order to better revere them?

Let us return to the more properly scientific aspects of the recent advances in the biology of the nervous system and the understanding of the mechanisms that control its development. It must be said that one of the major characteristics of the nervous system is no doubt its plasticity. The brain cannot be considered as a network of permanently established cables, and cerebral aging as the result of an increasing number of units in this circuit being disconnected from the network and going out of operation. Although not positively demonstrated except in a few experimental models, it can be assumed that every day new nerve fibers are growing, synapses are becoming undone and new ones are being formed. These changes in the neuronal and, of course, glial landscape mark our adaptation, our capacity for learning and improvement which will continue until an advanced age and, in fact, until death.

Now it also appears that the mechanisms which control this plasticity in the adult are similar in part to the ones operative in embryonal development. In particular, certain growth factors responsible for the maturation of neurons also remain present in the adult organism, where they are involved in the maintenance and plasticity of the nervous system. As a consequence, all the research that has been conducted for many years on the embryogenesis of this system is of fundamental importance for understanding adult life and aging. This has suddenly led to the creation of a new branch of knowledge—gerontology—which preempts an important part of scientific activity. This interest in the aging of the brain is of course related to the infinite hope aroused by the prospects of retaining a "young" brain throughout life and especially of having the means to combat degenerative disorders such as Alzheimer's disease. Indeed, if we can understand the mechanisms of cerebral blood flow, of neuronal survival and plasticity, if we can master the techniques of transplantation, a new field of therapy will open up and the tools of a new pharmacology will be developed.

We touched above on the difficulty of human applications and the necessity of first developing animal models in order to minimize insofar as possible the risk to patients of such experimentation on humans. We have not mentioned the problem that such application poses from the standpoint of the very organization of scientific research. In the final chapter of this book, I shall come back to the distinction that must be made between basic research and applied research and to the question of the difficult but necessary relationship between these two areas.

DEVELOPMENTAL GENES AND QUESTIONS OF EVOLUTION

Before we do so, however, let us consider another illustration of the possible application of the data from developmental neurobiology and, more generally, from the genetics of development. We are no longer concerned just with the fallout of such discoveries for society, but with concrete action in another scientific field, evolution. Indeed, it is not impossible that the recent discoveries we have just described may provide us with the ability to create new breeds and even new species. There is much to reflect upon from the standpoint of theory pertaining to the mechanisms of evolution and also in economic terms since some of these species may be useful or attractive to humans.

We should add that in some ways, empirically speaking, this ability is not entirely new. Gardeners and breeders have long since found ways to create, if not new species, at least new varieties and breeds of great interest to humans through the use of genetic selection, even without being aware of it. But the discovery and study of developmental genes have completely changed the equation.

From a theoretical standpoint, the question of the evolution of species is seen in a new light. In particular, it appears that we are now in a position to intervene in the dispute that has arisen in recent years with respect to the change that occurs when passing from one species to another: is it the result of a slow process of accumulation, over very long geological periods, of small variations subject to selection, as classical Darwinism would have it, and also more recently the synthetic theory of evolution (Ernst Mayr)? In other words, should we consider that passing from one species to another by way of interspecies evolution, occurs on the model of evolution within a species, or "intraspecies evolution"? Or should we conclude, along the lines suggested by Stephen Jay Gould and his school, that it is an abrupt passage due to very rapid events?

Let me briefly review the terms of the problem. Charles Darwin himself, in the 19th century, was well aware that one of the major obstacles to his theory of natural selection lay in the arrangement of the fossils as they were discovered in geological strata. Darwinian theory assumed that between two different forms related in a direct filial line there had to be every intermediate form that one could expect as a result of small variations. However, examination of geological strata has failed to uncover such intermediate forms.

There are two possible explanations for this: either we assume that these intermediate forms disappeared as a result of catastrophic events that have marked the history of the Earth, or that such intermediate forms never existed in fact and that the passage from one species to another occurs without transition.

We need not dwell on the classical hypothesis, to which many specialists still subscribe. Gould and his school maintain that interspecies evolution is abrupt. How do they explain it? We can conceive, they say, that at a particular point in the evolution of a species there appears—locally as a result of a few mutations, in a microenvironment—a different species that will develop on its own in that isolate. Under those conditions, the two species—the one that produced the new species and the new species itself—coexist in different territories with different sexual habits of reproduction and therefore without interbreeding.

Let us now suppose that some geological catastrophe, such as the sea receding, or the movement of glaciers, results in the disappearance of the first species that had been the more far-ranging and numerous of the two. And let us also suppose that for reasons related precisely to the conditions of the isolate, only the new species survives, sheltered from the catastrophe, for example in a pond that continues to exist while all the water in the surrounding area has receded. That species would remain there confined in a highly selective and localized environment for as long a period as we care to imagine. But let us also suppose that the water returns in the next period marked by the melting of the ice. At that point, the species preserved in its isolate would have free reign. It would no longer be in competition with the individuals from the first species who would all have disappeared; it could therefore extend its territory on a mass scale and develop.

When, hundreds of thousands of years later, we come to observe the geological strata, we find to our surprise that one species was suddenly and completely replaced by another. If we remain true to the classical theory, we will have to suppose that a very long time elapsed between the appearance of each form and that there had also been intermediate forms which, as we said, had vanished. Gould suggests that there was no considerable time lapse with respect to the formation of the new species, even if, as we have just seen, it took a long time and some major events before the new species was able to supplant the previous one completely.

It appears that this hypothesis can be supported by the discovery of developmental genes. Since these genes control the pattern of the organism as a whole rather than some minor characteristics (for example, eye color or hairiness), it is obvious that the mutation of one of these genes can play an important role in evolution by abruptly causing a very different organism to appear. That thesis was supported as early as 1940 by Richard Goldschmidt in the United States; he called such mutants "hope-bearing monsters." He was ridiculed by a number of his colleagues for his hypothesis that these monsters could emerge very quickly, "practically overnight."

We must not jump from one extreme to the other; this hypothesis needs to be confirmed experimentally. But it is one of the most exciting prospects in developmental genetics. Let us suppose that we discover genes whose expression plays a part at some given moment in the size of a particular organ or of a particular region of the nervous system; let us further suppose that we are able to control the expression of this type of gene and to implant it in an egg; we could then conceivably *experiment with evolution*. The fact is that given all those conditions, we could create new species, not by gradually selecting specific traits, but by producing within a given species the expression of genes from a different species. This would drastically alter the status of the theory of evolution; it would fall under Sir Karl Popper's definition of refutable theoretical scientific concepts; evolutionism would become an experimental science.

The technical procedure would be one of gene transfer: a gene is inserted in an egg which is then reimplanted in an animal to observe the direct effect of the presence of that gene; but it is also possible to prevent the expression of a gene that is normally present or to change the period during which it is expressed, in order to observe what happens. These genetic experiments—or genetic manipulations or genetic engineering, as some wish to call it—will make it possible (as is already the case) to observe in these transgenic animals the role of a given gene in the normal development of an individual.

Of course, one of the prerequisites for such gene transfers would be to determine which genes could affect development or distinguish one species from another fairly closely related one. Such detailed knowledge is not yet available but is within reach. The program recently adopted by international research organizations which involves mapping the entire human genome constitutes for our species a step toward achieving this dream.

Let us now suppose that through the use of such techniques we are able to create a new individual with reproductive functions. This would open the door to the rational creation of new breeds and even new species.

In the near future, some major areas of neurobiology will probably be developed. First, we will have to establish the basic rules for developmental formation, that is to say, the plans of the cerebral organ, which are identical within a given species but vary from one species to another. We would wager that this approach, with its genetic facet, will open the way to an understanding of interspecies evolution. Once these rules have been deciphered, we will have to understand the mechanisms by which they are implemented. Thus, we will have to study the regulation of the expression in space and time of the molecules that control the division, death, migration, and differentiation (including lineage) of the cells that compose the brain.

A second facet of this research is concerned with understanding the role played by nervous activity in the epigenetic constitution of the cerebral structure. Within a genetically determined package, the number of neurons, the form of the networks, and the number and distribution of the synapses reflect the history of the individual and the activity of his or her nervous system. Therefore, we can say that, in its details, the development of the brain is not governed by any automatism or inevitable force (except that of the sensory, affective or cultural environment). Therefore, what we have to establish and couple with the data supplied by the behavioral sciences is a science of functional embryology.

Of course, the points we have mentioned briefly and, we hope, simply, cannot be considered separately from each other. For example, we know that the location of a cell within cellular tissue influences its developmental choices.

Finally, we should make it clear that no one has a right to limit the scope of what may become possible, and that tomorrow some new branch of science may prove promising and start to develop, even though our arbitrary mental dissection may have failed to allow the necessary room for it. That such an unpredictable necessity should appear on the horizon is not something to be feared but rather to be desired.

THE PHILOSOPHICAL AND POLITICAL REPERCUSSIONS OF RESEARCH

INDIVIDUALITY

Of course, all the research and output of new knowledge just described has major philosophical repercussions which, in turn, entail considerable social and political consequences.

Let us consider from this angle one of the dominant themes that runs through this book. If what we have stated is correct, we can hypothesize that the higher a species stands along the evolutionary scale, the greater the importance of the epigenetic as opposed to the genetic component in the developmental formation of individuals.

Look at the bee as a classic example: even though its behavior is extraordinarily sophisticated, as people have often noted with admiration, this sophistication essentially is not based on individual learning; rather, it has been regulated during the course of evolution by a genetic constraint in the organization of its neuronal circuits. Under those conditions, no extrapolation from the bee to vertebrates makes any sense. Speculations by certain ethologists with sociobiological leanings who believe that conclusions based on societies of bees can be applied to human societies are unfounded, for a very simple reason that often passes unnoticed: the very notion of the individual has a different meaning among bees and among vertebrates. Let us be clear on this point: the idea of an animal society is not absurd *per se*, but we have to understand very precisely what this term encompasses and we must avoid the mechanical application of a scientific analysis valid for bees to the organization of other societies, and in particular to societies of vertebrates.

Since the epigenetic and the genetic components are never the same from one species to the next, the reality of the individual is likewise different in each case. Therefore, we cannot assign the same meaning to the term individual when we speak of a bee and, let us say, a beaver, to take another animal popular in fables.

But let us come back to the case of the human animal, the one in which we are ultimately interested. If we believe that the theory of evolution is a scientific one and not some idle speculation, as some people still believe today when they put it on the same level as the biblical story of Genesis, we must admit that there is a historical and genealogical link between some so-called lower primates and humans. There is nothing fundamentally different between *Homo sapiens* and its less evolved ancestors like the chimpanzee. In fact, if we analyze the genetic difference between humans and chimpanzees, we find that, quantitatively speaking, it is extremely small. For what such estimates are worth, it has been estimated at approximately one percent of the entire genome. But there is reason to believe, again based on recent discoveries, that many of these different genes belong to the category of developmental genes, including in particular but not exclusively some that may be involved in the development of certain regions of the central nervous system, for example the frontal cortex or the language areas.

This idea that the difference between us and our ancestors is partly a result of mutations affecting development is actually not completely new. It had been put forward, in another form of course, by many investigators since the 1920s. In those days, they used the notion of neoteny, meaning the persistence in the sexually mature adult of prepubertal traits. For example, De Beer used to say that humans were nothing but neotenic chimpanzees. He meant that human adults, capable of reproducing sexually, have many points in common with the embryonal chimpanzee, but that development has gone further in the chimpanzee whereas in humans it has stopped at the embryonic stage. Thus, hairiness in humans resembles that of the chimpanzee embryo, as does the position of the foramen magnum, the position of the vagina, the nonopposition of the thumb (great toe) to the other digits in the lower extremities, etc.

To translate this into modern terms, mutations that slow the rate and reduce the duration of expression of certain developmental genes may be responsible for the creation of traits distinguishing the human species from certain primates. Therefore, there is no reason to believe that the human species is fundamentally different from the others; the results of these studies certainly go in the direction of a materialism of sorts.

But I must underscore the fact that recent scientific developments enable us to understand what an individual is; they show that this very notion takes on different meanings depending on the species. The more limited the determination due to the strictly genetic component as contrasted with the epigenetic factors, the more the very structure of the nervous system is thereby linked to the history of the individuals. In other words, two individuals who have exactly the same genetic content will be virtually identical in bees; they will be very different in humans.

The central nervous system in humans forms a sort of engram of our personal histories; and the human individual who is unique and therefore not clonable is the result of a social history. In bees, all individuals are practically (but undeniably not quite) clones. Two humans, even if absolutely identical genetically, are never clones because the history of each individual remains singular from birth to death. That history is marked in the physical structure, including even in the cerebral matter itself, because of the importance of epigenesis which stabilizes a particular circuit or another. And if language, which obviously is basic to the humanity of our species, is linked to the structure of a particular area of the brain, to its synaptic conformation, to the number of cells that constitute it and to any other epigenetic trait, the language of an individual ties in with the process of his or her individuation: with the affective history, mental history, and history of the individual's interactions with other individuals in society.

The human individual is therefore an extreme individual; and at the same time an extremely social individual; at once the most individual and the most social of animals; the most individual by reason of being, by nature, the most social. These facts, it seems to me, make it possible for us to reconsider on a new basis the discussions on the innate and the acquired (nature and nurture) that had often started off badly.

As an example, let us take up a burning issue. I am convinced that the developmental perspective we have just outlined can reduce, if not completely eliminate, the hostility between neurobiologists, or those known as biological psychiatrists, and the mainstream psychoanalysts, to whatever school they may belong.

When biologists describe behavioral disorders (neuroses, psychoses) as being inscribed in the neuronal structure of the brain, psychoanalysts interpret this in the wrong way and imagine that it refers to something innate. They are convinced that people maintain that there is *ipso facto* for example a gene for schizophrenia or obsessive-compulsive neurosis and that the disease automatically affects any individual who carries that gene.

We must concede to them that, on the basis of genealogical data demonstrating a hereditary component for certain forms of mental illness, there have been ideologues who have tried to generalize and to exploit the results of researches in molecular biology to support such *radically and exclusively geneticist* aberrations, who are always on the verge of being criminal. Remember the first lobotomies!

On this question, there is a profound misunderstanding. The position of serious neurobiologists is simply that most of these behaviors are related to certain structuralizations of the neuronal networks; this in no way means that such behaviors are innate or unavoidable because of some genetic component. On the contrary, it is conceivable that they are structures which were formed during the development of the individual and have become stabilized as a result of the affective environment that the individual had to confront in the course of his or her unique history. From this perspective, a neurotic psychic structure may actually correspond very well to a neuronal network structure.

We will take the chance of clashing a little more with the idealist convictions of most psychoanalysts by encroaching resolutely on their domain. Is it not possible that analysis works through a change in the neuronal networks which is achieved painfully through transference during the recollection of childhood memories, since we know that in humans the neurons remain plastic until an advanced age, if not throughout life? If we are able some day to visualize some of these whole networks, for instance by means of new medical imaging techniques, perhaps we will be able to come to a definite conclusion. I like to think that during an analysis session we will be able to see a change in certain networks and the untying of certain "knots" we could call (why not?) "neurotic knots." There is nothing in this that seems to me outrageous from the standpoint of neurobiology. Why should psychoanalysts take offense? Would Freud himself have rejected this hypothesis?

As for drugs used by psychiatrists, it is somewhat too facile to reject them out of hand, as some opponents of psychiatry did in the past in the name of an existentialist-tinged philosophy. Some people went too far in using the term chemical strait jacket, even though they were right in denouncing certain excesses which even today are unfortunately too common. There is no doubt that where these substances interfere with the neuronal networks and alter their activity, they can prove effective. Tomorrow's problem will be to proceed on the basis of a more precise understanding of the networks, that is, to replace empirical medicine by scientific knowledge insofar as possible, in order to develop new drugs with more refined and precise applications to treat that type of disorder, but of course only in those cases where the disorder is troublesome to the individual concerned.

More than this, we hope that through pharmacological refinements we will be able to produce pleasurable sensations or intellectual stimulations without damage to the individual. In the name of what morality should psychotropic drugs used on a mass scale have to be limited to "socializing" substances such as Valium and other benzodiazepines?

There is a new conclusion to be drawn from this concept of the human individual as the extreme social individual: we must reconsider the relative position of the human species with respect to other species. Provided that we can expurgate it from all the theological meanings that have been associated with it in the past, I believe that it is possible and necessary to use the notion of a scale. From our angle, there is indeed a real scale of species, a real evolutionary scale.

Let us not forget that the human animal goes through the longest period of learning in relation to its average lifespan. We know that in humans the development of the central nervous system continues on to an advanced age. Human beings probably retain throughout their lives a very great capacity for plasticity. Some day, this plastic capacity may be increased further through human engineering. We know that closure of the cranial sutures is not final until between the ages of 15 and 20, which, nowadays in the developed countries, is equivalent to about a fourth of a human life! We should add that humans have one of the largest brains in comparison with the other bodily organs. Finally, let us remember that the cerebral areas associated with cognitive and mental functions are the most developed in the animal kingdom.

If we believe that greater value is to be placed on having the language and cognitive areas more developed than the olfactory areas, we can say that humans are "higher" on the scale than the dog, for example. Of course, this is our own assessment; we, the beings with the developed cortex, are the ones who establish the scale. It has no value *per se*, independently of the judgments we make. Thus, we can also say, without any fear of contradiction, that so far as evolution is concerned, a bee is as perfect as a chimpanzee.

There is another aspect of these researches whose philosophical implications should be underscored and given thought: the relationship between sexuality and reproduction.

As François Jacob expressed it in *La Logique du vivant* [The logic of the living], one of the great steps in the history of species was the invention of sexual reproduction. Whereas previously, one cell made two cells ("a cell's dream: to make another cell"), from the time sexual reproduction was "invented," it took two individuals to make one. And since sexual reproduction allows multiple chromosomal combinations, the children are of course very different from the parents and very different from each other.

It appears today that the second very significant invention of evolution was to separate, in humans, the reproductive functions and the sexual functions. While in most species sexuality and reproduction virtually overlap, the human species makes the greatest distinction between the two. To be sure, sexuality is part of a general reproductive process, and in a recent book, Jean-Didier Vincent (*Biologie des passions* [The biology of passion], Odile Jacob, 1986) presents a very good analysis of the hormonal mechanisms that underlie orgasm during copulation; he shows that pleasure is related to the activity of cerebral structures in the hypothalamus. But the structure involved in fantasizing, the one that can control this hormonal machinery, in particular, is linked to the cortex of the individual and hence, as I mentioned before, to the history of the individual, unique in each case, which is inscribed in the cortex. The result is a multiplicity of possible pleasures unrelated to the reproductive function. The body can respond to this multiplicity in a thousand ways, all of them individual, according to an infinity of scenarios; for our purposes, it is irrelevant to what extent, if any, these ways and scenarios may in all cases be consistent with a social code. The reader may consult his or her own experience or give free rein to the imagination.

What I would like to emphasize, however, as a matter of scientific objectivity of obvious emancipatory value, is that any morality seeking to link reproduction and sexuality in human beings is a morality more applicable to monkeys. God knows, there are such doctrines, and some are among the most rigid in our Christian Western world. And yet, this invention of sexuality for its own sake, which is exclusive to the human species, is no doubt related to the exceptional potential for fantasizing and cognition of the human brain. The arts, the sciences, and thought in general are the fruits of this marvelous invention.

Freud, who perhaps is not read enough by the biologists, wrote some very beautiful passages in his early works on the biological substrate of mental phenomena, and in particular on how energy passes from one cell to the next. In his *Entwurf einer Psychologie* [Outline of a Scientific Psychology] he even invented, if not the term, at least the concept of synaptic facilitation. The points he develops are far from being off the mark from the standpoint of current biological theory. To borrow and transpose an apt phrase coined by Canguilhem, let us say that he was "in the right," even if in those days they did not have the conceptual instruments or biological knowledge necessary to state what is right. But independently of these technical aspects of biological research which he never resigned himself to abandon, no matter what some people may say, I believe that the dissociation between reproduction and sexuality in humans which he himself established in his famous theory of drives and his concept of the libido, is fully in accord with the researches described in these pages. He was right in wanting to broaden, as he put it, the notion of sexuality by freeing it from its narrowly genital sense.

Freudian views aside, we believe that in any event it can be maintained that any structure, familial or otherwise, which claims that reproduction is the purpose of sexuality and presents this purpose as natural is invoking nature in vain. If indeed we require some foundation for this purpose, it is not in the natural order that we must look for it but in the social order. This order, of course, will generate more disputes, but is it right to deny conflicts by resorting to the fiction that the basis is to be found in nature? In any event, science cannot participate in fabricating such fiction.

SCIENTIFIC RESPONSIBILITY

When I referred earlier to the fact that it would eventually be possible to create new species through genetic engineering, for example by gene transfer, I was of course touching upon one of the most sensitive points of philosophical and political discussions that have accompanied recent developments in our branch of science. It is said, often with solemnity, that such investigations, like other no doubt better known ones with embryos, raise ethical questions. Since, as I understand it, these debates appeal to principles, I may be permitted here to defend a position likewise based on principle.

Ethics, as conceived of today, particularly through its "machinery," those well-known ethics committees, is essentially in the hands of physicians and jurists, even if they are sometimes joined by philosophers and members of the clergy of different faiths. But exactly on what basis are those persons entitled to lay down the law as regards relationships between the state and the individual? A serious question, indeed, because it involves no less than the concept and exercise of democracy in these matters.

It is true that we are now able to accomplish what only yesterday was barely thinkable but not achievable. The fact is that the development of the biological sciences is providing us with new knowledge which, if it clears the steps leading to applications, can have a major social impact, for example on our concepts of filiation, or descendency, and the fabric of law pertaining to it. There are two points on which we must be clear: although it is perfectly legitimate to prohibit certain applications, under no circumstances must such prohibition ever have the effect of choking off new knowledge. Application is one thing but the acquisition of new knowledge is another, with its own ethics, namely, to be infinite, by its very nature incomplete and unfinished, and by right unfinishable. Let us not mince words: this is the very foundation of great thought.

As for choosing whether or not a particular application ought to be tried or should be prevented, that is not the responsibility of scientists. This choice must be made by society and, I repeat, it cannot be left to the decision of two or three committees, no matter how distinguished their members or how pluralistic their composition. It is admittedly a choice which, under the present conditions of society cannot be made satisfactorily, for it would require an enlightened citizenry capable of understanding the issues at stake. Unfortunately, such is not the case. That is why it is urgent that a policy for spreading scientific culture be implemented by all available means to reinforce the basic knowledge acquired in school. France, the country of enlightenment, should lead the way and stop relying on models of expertise imported from across the Atlantic that are based on a different philosophy and another way of implementing policy, whose limitations and difficulties are recognized even by those directly concerned.

I would not want these general considerations on democratic decision-making to be taken as a profession of faith that has no specific or immediate application in the field of research discussed in this book. Two current examples will show that the opposite is true. The first raises a question which is the subject of public speeches and controversies. The second involves taboos, that is to say, questions that are avoided in speeches and evaded in discussions.

The first example is one that touches us very directly as researchers, since it has to do with the use of human embryos as a source of material for cell transplants, for example neurons. As mentioned earlier, once all preliminary experiments have been done as extensively as is necessary in laboratory animals, it will be possible to consider grafting embryonic cells in humans. For this purpose, human embryos would be more appropriate than rat or pig embryos. From a technical standpoint, there are no insurmountable difficulties in taking cells from embryos obtained from therapeutic abortions or even from embryos produced for the sole purpose of serving as organ banks.

The question that arises is not technical in nature but rather ethical or even philosophical. Of course, it raises the whole problem of the development of a market in embryos, similar to the market in babies for adoption that has recently developed.

The issues that are being questioned here concern both social organization and the embryo's potentially human status. Scientists are not qualified to make decisions alone any more than is any other segment of society. There is only one way a democratic decision can be made: it must follow a public debate in which every facet of the question is examined, making it possible to draw up legislation that takes into account the interests of science and medicine, the requirements of society, the convictions of the majority of its citizens and the rights of minorities.

The other example is very different; it concerns the possibility of manufacturing drugs that would not be injurious to health and would give individuals pleasurable sensations that they would be free to enjoy. We can see the advantage of developing such products: the death-dealing traffic in today's illicit drugs would be compromised. But would they have to be marketed or even, in some cases, distributed free of charge? Here, too, the decision will have to be based on profound democratic reflection and cannot be left to some committee of specialists, no matter who they are.

If such an exercise in democracy could come to be, I personally would wish that attention should not be focused solely and obsessively as it is today on genetic engineering, which is made into a cheap bugbear, while we ought not to forget that it also offers immense hope for the treatment of the most terrible diseases. I would like attention also to be paid to the biggest engineering of them all, the one that is practised every day, in the good conscience of people worldwide, namely, the epigenetic engineering or manipulation of children through education, the press, radio, and television, not to mention the selling of children or malnutrition, etc., whose terrible reality is brought to our attention periodically through some ringing reports issued by international organizations.

For that matter, we might wonder how this obsession concerning the ownership of the embryo came about in the first place. There is no doubt that in addition to humanitarian concerns, with which we can all agree, there were other motivations in the definition given by the French government's Council of State in a report on these questions relating to what it called "the natural structures of parenthood." Among these other concerns, we can clearly see a defense of the prevailing morality, the hereditary transmission of property, etc.

You may ask me whether I do not approve of the spectacular action taken by Professor Jacques Testard who decided to stop his research because of problems of conscience that he had with *in vitro* fertilization and the implantation of embryos in surrogate mothers. I respect all decisions dictated by problems of conscience, but my answer is that I do not approve of the action taken by Professor Testard; and I worry about the interpretations that may be put it. Does it not suggest a terrible confusion between basic research and applied research? The question raised by this confusion is whether or not we feel that, in a society such as ours, the function of producing new knowledge is one that we intend to maintain independently of all possible applications. Testard has discontinued his research: clearly, he believes that anything that may lead to applied research is potentially, if not already, applied research; to his mind, the difference between basic research and applied research is only a question of degree. This is a deplorable idea, suggesting that there can be no research with purely cognitive intent, that such research is illegitimate from a societal standpoint, and that basic science is haunted by or, if you prefer, infested with some sort of inevitability of application. That idea did not spring up suddenly, like mushrooms after a downpour; it has in fact been making headway for many years, and not only in biology; in the past, in nuclear physics, it appeared in a leftist and revolutionary guise and today is expressed in the language of puritan humanism.

I think it is absolutely vital to remind ourselves that there is a legitimate distinction between basic and applied research; that is of course true even if we are called upon to engage in basic research knowing full well from the very outset that it may ultimately lead to applications. But depending on the particular case, the research aspect is not the same. In our own field, let us take a futuristic example, almost in the realm of science fiction, to clarify this crucial point. As we have explained, it may be possible some day to create new species thanks to the discovery of developmental genes and the gene transfer techniques we have described. It would then be conceivable to take a chimpanzee, for example, and modify its cognitive faculties. At that point, there might be industrial executives who would become interested in the research, thinking that such creatures could make excellent robots for building machines or automobiles. From the standpoint of a free-market economy for the production of goods, they would have neither the disadvantages of humans nor those of robots and could combine the qualities of both. These industrialists would then contact the laboratory and tell the researchers: try to build us some chimpanzees with such and such characteristics, to work on a production line! In this setting, the research, which still remains research, obviously takes on a different aspect.

And how should scientists respond? As scientists, they will say neither yes nor no. But as citizens, they may well have opinions; it is as citizens that they will lean in favor of a choice that is not a scientific one but, in the strictest sense of the term, a political one. Suppose that the answer were positive and that in their hearts and souls they are horrified, would they have to suspend all research on the evolution of the nervous system? As we can see, that distinction between a basic and sometimes unexpected discovery and a planned, rational, and determined application has more than just theoretical implications. It makes it possible to designate the area in which the democratic debate should take place with regard to the societal consequences of the decision to proceed or not to proceed with the application.

Does that mean that scientists have no responsibility? Far from it. First, they have to acquire the data and submit the quality of their findings to the scientific community. In France, there are scientific commissions at INSERM (National Institute of Health and Scientific Research) and the CNRS (National Scientific Research Center) that fulfill this function. Members elected by the personnel and appointed by the directors of the organizations constitute "research parliaments" which, on the whole, do their jobs very well. In fact, every country has its specific form of control, usually through the scientists' own peers. In the United States, for example, the judgments are made when the researchers are hired by a university or when research funds are allocated. In the case of medical research, committees at the National Institutes of Health on which scientists sit, judge the quality of the projects, and decide whether subsidies should be granted.

Another responsibility of scientists is to inform the public and warn political organizations of the possible consequences of some particular application. They thereby create the conditions for the exercise of democracy and make sure that military, economic or other pressure groups do not impose decisions regarding applications, made in secret or, rather, in ignorance. To develop a true scientific culture is increasingly becoming a democratic imperative in which scientists are duty-bound to participate.

Finally, it is up to scientists to learn how to mobilize and coordinate their research efforts on an international scale when there is an urgent need to do so for humanitarian reasons. At the same time, they have a duty to alert the decision-makers and opinion-makers as to the exact nature of the peril and the legitimate fears that it may cause; they must also reject demagoguery, which is disastrous in this context, not yield to the temptation of premature announcements, resist fostering unrealistic expectations or raising false hopes, even though in the short term that may bolster irrational fears.

It seems to me that the recent viral epidemic responsible for AIDS—a disease that affects not only the immune system but also, as I will explain in closing, the central nervous system in dramatic proportions, causing more or less extensive destruction of the patient's cognitive faculties—is a striking example of the ability of the scientific and medical community to mobilize on a mass scale. Developmental neurobiology is contributing to the common effort to understand this scourge and curb its progress.

We should point out that the very rapid advances made in describing the infectious agent, which will eventually make it possible to develop vaccines and treatments, could not have been achieved without the conceptual potential of the most scientifically developed countries. Ultimately, it is thanks to basic research and to the knowledge accumulated as a result of these efforts without being concerned with applications that the information gathered was able to be used as a whole in necessary and urgent research directed toward a specific end.

However, this epidemic calls for some very serious thinking of a different kind. We are entitled to wonder why certain of the most prominent figures in the medical field, including some who sit on ethics committees whose role it is to consider such issues, failed to exercise their moral prerogative to demand, back in 1985, that a policy of prevention be established. Why did it take so long to launch large-scale information campaigns, why has there been a delay in permitting the unrestricted sale of syringes and condoms?

Let us not mince words: at a time when the scientific and medical community was mobilizing, the politicians and the people in the media, who usually are quick to demand ever greater economic productivity from the work of researchers, remained virtually silent with their arms folded. No doubt in order to avoid offending the moral majority, they thus sent to a certain death thousands of persons throughout the world, most of them drug addicts, homosexuals, convicts, and Africans.

But let us drop this point. History, which unfortunately is moving very rapidly in this area, has already made a judgment. We had better get back to the question of the relationship between basic research and research directed to specific purposes, which is so difficult to establish on a sound basis.

THE ORGANIZATION OF RESEARCH

Basic research and, in particular, neurobiology so far as we are concerned constitute a fund of knowledge whose development for concrete applications would have considerable social and financial implications. The social implications, which we need not discuss again, include, besides the question of AIDS, the previously mentioned importance of degenerative diseases and the aging of the nervous system. The financial implications are obvious: we need only think of the profits to be made by the pharmaceutical companies that first develop and market these drugs of the future.

However, this industrial development requires considerable investment and know-how and raises the political question of the relationship between basic research and applied research. Let me briefly elaborate on a few of the points that touch on this serious question.

First of all, the primary mission of basic research is to produce new knowledge that may, though not necessarily, be directed to specific ends. Therefore, we cannot reduce basic research without eventually depriving ourselves of the means of gaining understanding and knowledge, and if necessary of using its results for purposes that meet a social need. Next, the sector concerned with industrial and commercial exploitation must keep abreast of the very latest advances in research in order to be able to operate properly. This requires not only that its links with the public sector be improved, but that the private sector have its own basic research tools. Lastly, we know that applied research requires considerable capital outlay for the development of special technologies, feasibility tests, therapeutic trials, etc. We will cite precise examples to help us understand certain aspects of these problems.

The first of these points, that is, the impossibility of predicting the social fallout of any particular basic research effort, can be illustrated by the work done on *Drosophila*. Some people might scoff at scientists who are interested in the development of the fruit fly and the number of hairs (actually, sensory appendages of the nervous system) it has. And yet it was these researchers, spurred on by their curiosity to understand the genetic control mechanisms of morphogenesis through a simple model, who demonstrated the developmental genes we discussed earlier. We now know that those genes also exist in vertebrates, including humans, and that they are strongly expressed in the nervous system. There also, as in the fly, their function is to regulate gene expression. As a result, those genes, or rather the protein products that bind to the genome at specific sites, could become a target for new pharmacological agents. Practically all of the large pharmaceutical groups are already pointing their research in this direction.

Following the persistent focus on what may be considered as essential to human health (or more often to the health of the economy) by short-sighted decision-makers, some countries are dropping whole segments of research which, in spite of its absolute basic appearance, may unexpectedly be breeding fertile applications. Some day, those who are in charge of the future will have to accept this unpredictable aspect of research which by its very nature is beyond planning.

Actually, this story about *Drosophila* is no fable. We need only remember the arguments used by Trofim Denisovich Lysenko when he led the final attack against Soviet geneticists in 1948. He strongly derided those "reactionary intellectuals" who, following the example of the bourgeois geneticists in the West, concerned themselves with the genetics of *Drosophila* and the number of hairs on this insect rather than thinking about improving species of animals or plants that are useful to humans, such as cows or corn. We know what happened to Soviet genetics, at the time among the world's best in the field, and ultimately to Soviet agriculture, which is still paying the price for the biological disaster of the Lysenko years.

So, let us be wary of any creeping Lysenkoism, because Lysenkoism was not simply one individual's folly or a hoax of Marxist philosophy he spouted, but also reflected the ideology of highly rationalist technocrats who wanted to bend the scientific process to their economic "emergencies."

Does this mean that we have to keep a basic science sector pure and free of any contact with the applied sector? No, of course not.

As we said before, the contacts between basic research and applied research must be expanded. For example, by motivating and helping industries to create their own basic research sector, we would be increasing at the same time the opportunities for interaction between those who have chosen basic research and those who have opted to work with an eye to scientific applications. It is even possible to envisage the creation of public applied research organizations that would be in close contact with other public organizations concerned with basic research. Even better, in view of the investments required, it should be considered normal practice for the government to finance part of the applied research, of course with controls over the use of public funds, as in the case of any public sector activity. What is less normal, or more disquieting, is the fact that when there is no research and development policy (there are, of course, exceptions), the private applications sector is increasingly dependent on the public basic sciences sector. A growing number of laboratories in the public sector could no longer survive without assistance from private industry and are forced to turn away from their own mission, which is to generate basic knowledge. We may wonder whether any basic research that has no "conceivable" application at the time of its conception is on its way to being doomed.

We should add this paradox: a good part of the money that public laboratories receive from private enterprise in this way is actually money that the government gives industry as an aid to develop research.

It is plain to see that this is an unhealthy process. It prompts companies to allocate only a small part of their total budget to the research and development of applications. At the same time, it allows them to use government money covertly to direct public research.

If the mongrel and confused system that we now have were to break away from the state of relative equilibrium in which it still maintains itself and to become completely unbalanced, we would witness a public research sector paid for with public funds, whose main activity would be to work on research projects of a practical nature imposed by private industry. In the long haul, make no mistake about it, this would lead to an impoverishment of the creative abilities of research as a whole, basic *and* applied.

We have a right to be fearful that this general ideological orientation, which does not specifically apply to any one country, will result in the disappearance of the prime motivation, or what ought to be the prime motivation, of those engaged in the professions of basic research: to create knowledge, to become intellectuals, and—why not?—even scholars.

This ideological orientation is to be found to an increasing degree even in the concrete way that research is organized, on the model of the ideology (some say the culture) of private enterprise. There is an extreme division of labor which, for certain types of research, is indeed a necessity, but which for others constitutes an impediment. As a result of this organization, a sort of standard career is emerging: a young researcher joins a laboratory. His or her first objective will be to write a thesis as soon as possible. During this period, the aim will be to produce as many results as possible. Then, the young researcher leaves for postdoctoral training, usually in another country, which in itself is a good thing. Upon returning, there will be a choice of three alternatives: set up one's own basic research laboratory, join an existing laboratory in a middle management position, or choose mobility by accepting a position in a corporate laboratory.

What can be expected from setting up one's own laboratory, that is to say, if the young researchers are among those endowed with the most outstanding qualities for research? Almost immediately, they will find themselves deep in administrative work to manage the division of labor; and those administrative tasks will gradually eat up the time that could have been devoted to research.

The key to success today is to know how to train and supervise young researchers. Far from resisting this trend, we go along with it. And of course this casual acceptance is legitimized by an ideological concept, according to which one has to be young to make discoveries. In fact, this simplistic concept derives from a common-sense, generally accepted idea, completely devoid of any biological basis and motivated by self-interest. As we pointed out earlier, the brain remains plastic until an advanced age. Perhaps some people will claim that if this notion has no biological basis, it may have a psychological or social basis. But for the few cases always mentioned of bright stars who have quickly burned themselves out, how many others much more impressive are there who have gone in the opposite direction? For instance, what would American research be today had it not been for the emigration of a generation of European Jewish researchers during the last world war? We should be aware of the fact that these researchers were not writing their theses: they were great veteran scientists who had long since made names for themselves. To mention only the neurosciences, a whole intellectual school was established in the United States through the impetus of Viktor Hamburger who carried on the work of Spemann; Rita Lévi-Montalcini, who worked in the United States for many years, owes an essential part of her Nobel prize to this school.

Our ideology really confuses scientific productivity, that is, the process of getting young researchers to perform the maximum amount of work in a brief period, and intellectual production itself. The latter can be achieved, for example, by choosing the right subjects for the young researchers to work on. And who are those who know how to choose the right subjects? They are people who have spent almost a lifetime in actual research, not in the administration of research, but people we call real scientists, who have an overall view of their field of science, who know its history and its prospects; those who can be said to have a scientific "sense": those who have an idea of where to look in order to make discoveries.

And yet, the model currently gaining ground in France, and more generally in Europe if not throughout the world, is tending, as I have said, to produce administrators exclusively on the one hand, and young researchers who are intensely but briefly productive, on the other. There may soon be a shortage of researchers capable of guiding this productivity toward the advancement of knowledge and whose experience allows productivity not to be limited to a fever of publications with no other goal than publishing for its own sake. In short, research needs scientific scholars.

THE MARCH OF SCIENTIFIC PROGRESS

Over the previous pages, we have succinctly tried to put into perspective the recent and, we hope, future advances of research on the development of the nervous system. Here we have indeed made some outstandingly spectacular progress. I am now coming back to this point not so much because of the concern I have just expressed regarding the organization of research, but rather to state my opposition to an increasingly pervasive ideology that feels entitled to cast the shadow of its political pessimism over scientific thought.

To show the advances that have been made, we concentrated on a particular structure as if were isolated: the structure of the central nervous system and, essentially, of the brain. Of course, this was a way of delimiting the subject, but no such natural limits exist. Indeed, the brain does not develop on its own, but, more particularly, according to sensory or external information. This means that insofar as its development is concerned, it is completely dependent on all the other organs of the body. And we could rightly say that a one-armed person does not think the same way as a person who has two hands.

More to the point, the nervous system is not isolated from other systems. For example, a great deal of emphasis is placed on the blood-brain barrier separating the brain from the rest of the organism which prevents the cells and even the proteins that are in the blood from penetrating freely into the cerebral matter; however, this barrier, as a result of the special way in which the cells that make up the blood vessel walls are organized, is extraordinarily porous. Thus, the brain is actually in contact with the entire organism through the sensory (afferent) fibers and the cerebral blood flow.

A revealing example of these contacts are the relationships between the nervous system and the immune system. These have been actively studied for some years. It has been observed in particular that mental states, such as depression for instance, affect the function of the immune system. It is known that recurrent attacks of herpes can often be precipitated by mental depression. It has also been known for a long time that a woman who is afraid of being pregnant will often experience delayed menstruation.

We know that there are cells belonging to the immune system in the brain itself: these include lymphocytes able to cross the blood-brain barrier and also what are called cerebral macrophages. There is considerable data indicating that these macrophages (cells generated in the bone marrow, outside the brain, that invade the brain during the development of the embryo) might differentiate into microglia. Those microglial cells mentioned in the first chapter qualify fully as cerebral cells and are therefore most probably, as regards their lineage, descendants of monocytic cells. After having crossed the blood-brain barrier during embryogenesis, they apparently acquire different properties, enabling them to participate in the physiology of the nervous system. They then synthesize proteins important for cerebral growth in that they stimulate the proliferation and maturation of astrocytes, and accelerate the formation of vessels and consequently the irrigation of the nervous system through the veins and arteries, which is obviously of fundamental importance for its proper operation.

It is not unreasonable to believe that these same microglia synthesize other factors that enable the neurons to survive or at least to function. Research has

112

now provided much evidence along those lines. One of the strongest indications that the cells help the neurons to function properly is the development of early dementia in certain AIDS patients, since the cells infected by the virus are essentially these microglial cells that are very probably derived from the immune system. It appears that infection of those cells by the virus has a significant effect on the cognitive functions themselves. This dramatic example is a very good illustration of the fact that interactions do exist between the two systems.

On a more conceptual level, the very mechanisms involved in the developmental formation of the nervous system may prove to be very similar to those involved in the development of the immune system. For example, when we speak of cell death and even of cell Darwinism, or of synaptic Darwinism, as is done today with regard to the specific survival of certain neurons or of certain networks, we are definitely drawing directly on models taken from immunology.

Here is another example of similarity and interdependence between the two systems: many molecules with a certain type of function in the immune system will be found in the nervous system, perhaps with functions of a different type. Hence, we cannot think of the brain as an isolated organ, either functionally or in its make-up, or even in the components and materials that constitute it. That is one of the major breakthroughs in neurobiology today; and reciprocally as well, in the areas of science interested in the other systems.

This theoretical situation is reflected by an ever-closer cooperation between the specialists in these two branches of research. The phenomena of adhesion, neuronal death and cell migration that we have briefly described also exist in the immune system. In that system, there is a class of cells, in particular, whose function is to kill other cells, and we are even beginning to understand how they operate. What we are discovering about the immune system may prove to be of invaluable help in understanding the workings of the nervous system.

In return, immunologists are using the work of neurobiologists to construct models for their own investigations. Those exchanges have given rise to a new and rapidly expanding branch of knowledge. The neurobiologists call it neuroimmunology and the immunologists call it immunoneurology: it depends from which side one looks at it or approaches it.

Let me use the development of neuroimmunology as a new discipline as an opportunity to take one last look at the conceptual history of the research which we have attempted to describe in this book.

In the first few pages, I spoke of the formulation of the concept of induction in 1930. Hans Spemann and Olivia Mangold had demonstrated the existence of an organizing center that neutralized the primitive ectoderm. Starting at that time, as I said, inductor research was on the agenda of many biology and especially biochemistry laboratories. The watchword soon became to combine biochemistry and embryology, and more broadly to merge genetics, embryology and evolution.

Those clarion calls were perfectly correct. However, for reasons they did not understand, even though they had the idea, the great scientists of the early part of this century, including G.R. De Beer, Jean Brachet, Richard Goldschmidt and Thomas Hunt Morgan, were unable to proceed further. They were not able to demonstrate that idea experimentally. This is a striking story, because before long there was the parallel development of another line of research in a completely different direction: molecular biology. But, in a sense, we can say that for quite a while, the lightning-fast development of molecular biology slowed the development of experimental embryology to an extraordinary degree—not because molecular biology was hostile to experimental embryology but because the events that were happening were so promising and so fascinating that young researchers were attracted to them in droves. We can now say that, in return, the progress of molecular biology made it possible to clear the obstacles that the experimental embryologists had encountered!

Therefore, a detour was necessary along a parallel avenue of research developing among the descendants of Pasteur's studies on microorganisms which had nothing to do with embryology, before embryology was able to resume its progress until, as we have noted, it joined with other disciplines such as neurology or evolution.

This is the way things happen in basic research: this detour was never thought out, nor planned by some strategist; under the conditions that existed at the time, it was not thinkable in those terms. We can see why a policy of planning for basic research is a dangerous trap. We may regret it, but the fact is that its avenues are essentially unpredictable and therefore impossible to plan. For my part, I believe that rather than regret this fact, we should be happy about it. That is what makes a calling devoted to intellectual adventure so fascinating.

BIBLIOGRAPHY

DE BEER, G.R.: *Embryos and Ancestors*, Clarendon Press, Oxford, 1958.

CANGUILHEM, G.: *Idéologie et Rationalité dans l'histoire des sciences de la vie* [Ideology and rationality in the history of sciences*], Vrin, Paris, 1977.

CHANGEAUX, J.P.: *L'Homme neuronal* [published in English as *Neuronal Man*, Oxford University Press, 1986], Fayard, Paris, 1984.

EDELMAN, G.M.: *Neural Darwinism. The Theory of Neuronal Group Selection*, Basic Books, Inc., New York, 1987.

GOULD, S.J.: *Ontogeny and Phylogeny*, The Belknap Press of Harvard University Press, Cambridge, Mass. and London, 1977.

GROS, F.: *Les Secrets du gène* [The secrets of the gene*], Odile Jacob, 1986.

JACOB, F.: *La Logique du vivant* [The logic of the living*], Gallimart, 1976.

JACOBSON, M.: *Developmental Neurobiology*, 2d ed., Plenum Press, New York and London, 1978.

MAYR, E.: *The Growth of Biological Thought: Diversity, Evolution and Inheritance*, Harvard University Press, Cambridge, 1982.

PROCHIANTZ, A.: *Les Stratégies de l'embryon* [Strategies of the embryo*], Presses Universitaires de France, 1988.

---

* These references have not been published in English.